I0502479

First, do no harm...Primum no nocere...

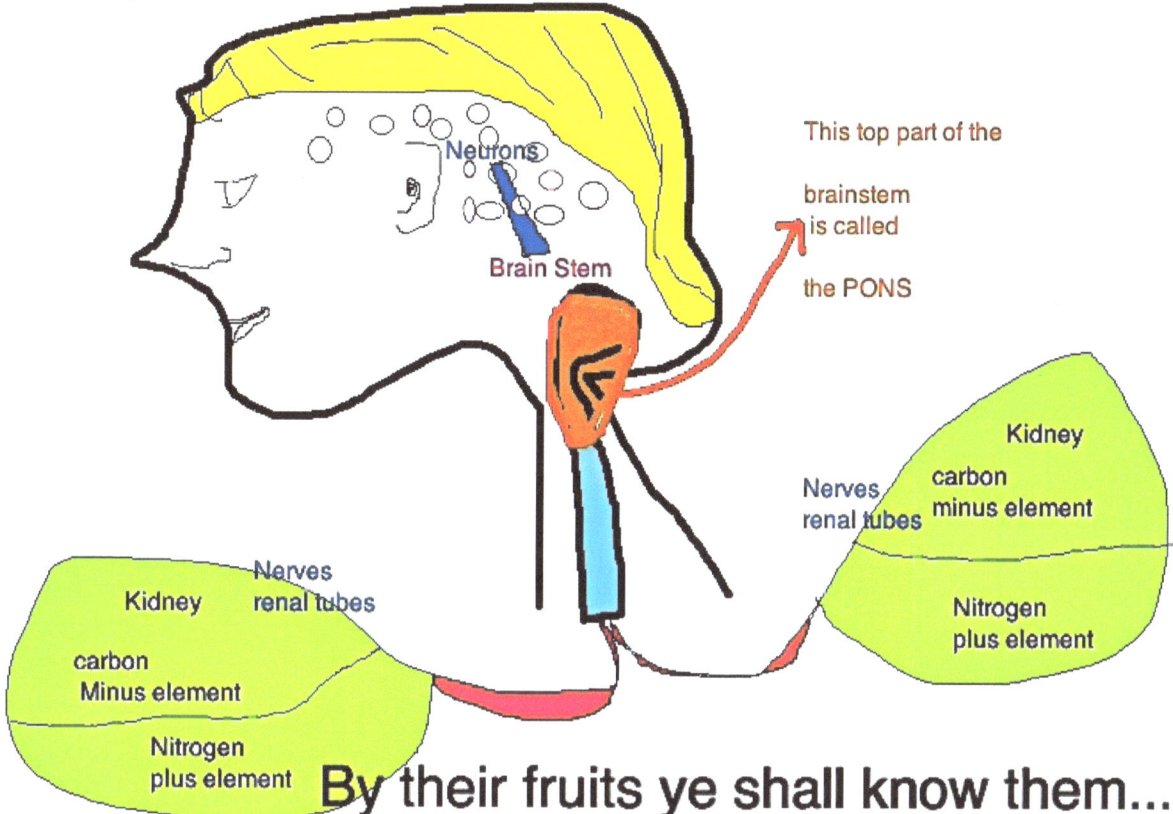

This top part of the brainstem is called the PONS

By their fruits ye shall know them...

A first comment about "First do no harm" (in Latin "Primum no nocere"):

The very first tenet(promise) of the Hippocratic oath(for physicians & surgeons) is First do NO harm...
 Not everybody takes this oath or promise...This is important to know...When in doubt, ask:"did you promise to first do no harm???"...Ask your doctor, the person running a clinical trial, the surgeon who is telling you facts, ask...
 Why?
 Because if they haven't they could be dangerous...
Dangerous? yes, dangerous...
At the very moment when a doctor is cutting into a rat on purpose to give it a disease, in order to run a clinical trial, that doctor has done harm...
At the very moment when a chimpanzee is given the Aids virus on purpose to study how it fights it, harm has been done first...
At the very beginning of any clinical trial, if a drug is given to people who do not need it, harm has been done...
Hurting someone on purpose is a violation of all that is noble & true in the Medical Arts, the art of healing...
Healers, artists of healing do not do harm first...

All those clinical trials where animals are harmed on purpose violate the basic tenet of the Hippocratic oath...
Those doctors participating in such trials are not doctors, they are outside of the licensing ethic of the greater body of Physicians & Surgeons...
Their practices are NOT acceptable according to medical ethics, & their licenses should be revoked...
Healing is an art...Harming is not an art...Know the difference...

New International Version James 4:10
Humble yourselves before the Lord, and he will lift you up.
http://biblehub.com/james/4-10.htm

Nelson Mandela(spoke of): "Ubuntu" (Humanness)
R.I.P. Thursday Dec.5, 2013 at around 5 pm Toronto time...
(Tuberculosis infections can occur when working in a prison quarry because cement is an Aluminum dust which gets into the lungs & later can get infected if it remains lodged there untreated...)

Do it yourself medicine:A repair manual
Copyright ©2014 by Joseph & Sari Grove
All rights reserved. No part of this
publication may be reproduced, stored in a retrieval system, or transmitted by any
means – electronic, mechanical,
photographic (photocopying), recording, or otherwise – without prior permission in writing
from the authors. Written in Canada,
Printed in South Carolina, U.S.A.
Paperback: 260 pages (this may vary with new updates & edits) Shipping Weight: 1.5 pounds
Product Dimensions: 11 x 8.5 x 0.6 inches
Learn more information at:
www.grovecanada.ca
3DIY Medicine:A Repair Manual by Joseph & Sari Grove ©2014 GroveCanada.ca
Publisher: CreateSpace Independent Publishing Platform (Note: New versions may be later than this: January 1st, 2014) Language: English ISBN-10: 1494392577
ISBN-13: 978-1494392574

Grove Body Part Chart Each Organ has a Minus Element & a Plus Element that must live in

Each Organ has 2 Opposing Elements...(Minus & Plus)

Organ	Minus Element	Plus Element
Thyroid	Zinc	Lead
Thymus	Manganese	Iron
Lungs & Lymph Nodes	Titanium	Aluminum
Heart	Potassium	Aurum
Kidneys	Carbon	Nitrogen
Pancreas	Selenium	Sulphur
Liver	Oxygen	Hydrogen
Adrenal Gland	Iodine	Calcium
Spleen	Copper	Phosphorus
Gallbladder	Magnesium	Mercury
Colon	Fluorine	Bismuth

Balance!

**Grove Body Part Chart:A medical arts innovation is our first book that deals with the chart, as seen below...You might want to read that book first to get the basic idea of how the chart works...This book Do it yourself medicine:A repair manual presupposes that you "get" the chart idea & moves into some ailments that are more complicated...

Grove Body Part Chart

Organ	Minus Element	Plus Element
Thyroid	Zinc	Lead
Thymus	Manganese	Iron
Lungs & Lymph Nodes	Titanium	Aluminum
Heart	Potassium	Aurum
Kidneys	Carbon	Nitrogen
Pancreas	Selenium	Sulphur
Liver	Oxygen	Hydrogen
Adrenal Gland	Iodine	Calcium
Spleen	Copper	Phosphorus
Gallbladder	Magnesium	Mercury
Colon	Fluorine	Bismuth

As a for example:If the book says bipolar is a Zinc excess in the Thyroid...Check the Chart...Lead is the Opposite element to Zinc...Check where to find Lead...Drink carrot juice daily as your personal treatment...

GROVE BODY PART CHART:A MEDICAL ARTS INNOVATION

GROVE BODY PART CHART

EACH BODY PART CONTAINS TWO ELEMENTS, THAT ARE OPPOSITES...

JOSEPH & SARI GROVE

ELEMENTS: where to find them

*Contents:These links are all clickable, if you are online...(all the way through)...

Home

Thyroid=Zinc(Minus element)+Lead(Plus element)

Thymus=Manganese(Minus element)+Iron(Plus element)

Lung & Lymph Nodes=Titanium(Minus element)+Aluminum(Plus element)

Heart=Potassium(Minus element)+Aurum(Plus element)

Kidneys=Carbon(Minus element)+Nitrogen(Plus element)

Pancreas=Selenium(Minus element)+Sulphur(Plus element)

Liver=Oxygen(Minus element)+Hydrogen(Plus element)

Adrenal Gland=Iodine(Minus element)+Calcium(Plus element)

Spleen=Copper(Minus element)+Phosphorus(Plus element)

Gallbladder=Magnesium(Minus element)+Mercury(Plus element)

Colon=Fluorine(Minus element)+Bismuth(Plus element)

(some)Social Networks for GroveCanada

About me: Sari Grove

The book, online, use the TRANSLATE feature to the far right of this blog to TRANSLATE the book...

OCT
8

1. Grove Body Part Chart

. (Some of these instructions are for only *If you visit our blog http://grovebodypartchart.blogspot.com online)

(*this is all if you are online)*To TRANSLATE this page or any other, please move your mouse cursor to the FAR RIGHT SIDE of this blog...HOVER OVER Those 3 slim black boxes...Choose the top one with the letter "A"...The word "TRANSLATE" pops up...

Click that to choose your language...Translate...

**(At the top LEFT of this Blog is the word PAGES...Go there, scroll to the bottom & you will see The BOOK online Page-click that-then you can TRANSLATE the book itself into your LANGUAGE...

Um:

(Um, you should know that my answers in my books are sometimes different from the online versions on our blogs, because the online versions are what I use to see & play around with my research ideas...The books are where I try to nail it down...I also edit & update the books if I see a mistake...Editing research, even if it is incorrect is dangerous because then you forget how you got somewhere, even if it was by mistake...So beware...You could die of a misprint! (that's a joke but sort of true!)

Also, if we are going to try the disclaimer route...I am a Canadian...Yes I am openly Canadian...Which means I am going to be looking more at problems I see here...Let's just say I am not as interested in suntanning rashes as frostbite numbness, & so on...

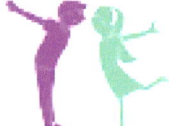

Joseph & Sari Grove (oh, my silent husband? He is the sub-text or the text depending on the day...But yes, if something sounds like a male thought it probably came from Joseph...Like he drinks beer, watches sports, & is not a huge fan of sushi...I love avocado, feeding Trumpeter swans(Cut Wheat, Cut Corn, Red Millet, White Millet, Black Oil Sunflower and Red Milo-these are the ingredients of Red Ribbon wild bird seed which is what I feed-a higher & more complex nutritional content than just corn, though I hear dog food kibble is even better for them than grains!) & well, generally speaking, we do line up along more traditional gender lines...Enough about that because gender typing is not my favorite subject...)(Been feeding them high energy bird suet for the Minus celsius days...The Trumpeter swans...But I digress...again...Suet has beef tallow in it which falls into the Aluminum cholesterol category on my chart...It raises cholesterol which is perfect for very cold winery

(I meant to write "wintery", but My Mum is in the wine business, a wine agent, owner of Lorac Wine inc., so I'm leaving that typo as a not so Freudian slip) days...

Beef tallow is in mincemeat pies too...For the same reason...Swans eat insects in the wild, which is a high protein thing...So don't get all huffy that suet is non-vegetarian...Insects are meat...)

One of the "saying" plates that was on the wall of my Mum's office:"Life is too short to drink cheap wine"...

Wine often contains alot of Nitrogen(In your Kidneys), which makes you smarter(though a little more hostile)...Wine grapes also contain Iodine, which lowers Cancer/Calcium levels in the Adrenal Gland...Cyanidins in grape skins are an Oxygen element on the Periodic Table of Elements, which dry out a wet liver that suffers from the mood called Depression or has the common cold...Hydrogen in wine is found in water, which is opposite to Oxygen in the Liver...Cheap wine usually has less of these...Unless it is family made Blueberry wine in Italy, & then it is free, but full of good stuff...(The best wine I have ever tasted was that, at VinExpo, a son of a winemaker let me try it-sneaky try...)

Lately:

Lately there is a lot of talk about vaccinations...To do or not to do...Basically it's like this...Mostly they help like most people alot of the time...Then there are this way smaller tinier group of people who got side effects...Those people had a bad time from vaccinations...So the answer is get informed...Figure out who exactly you are & what your vulnerabilities & strengths are...Then try to figure out which vaccine is which & what might be in it, & is the clinic clean or dirty, public or private, are the people nice or mean & too busy? Does their refrigerator look like it is running well & everything is cold enough?(A hot vaccine can come back to life if it is the cheaper variety sometimes found in poorer countries)...Short Answer:Get educated...Then apply that to your own life...If you have epilepsy, your children might be fluorine sensitive & tetanus shot sensitive so you may be walking into a disaster...Think about that before going in & state all those facts at the time of injection in case you missed a thought...A smart healthcare provider might send you home to think about it more & let you come back later if you still want it...

Like here are some things to consider:

You could become deaf from measles. (*deafness is in the Temporal Lobe & can be caused by Fluorine excess)...

Your child could be born with compromised eyesight from rubella...(**eyesight issues are in the Pancreas & can be caused by excess Sulphur, think sugars...)

You can get pneumonia from chickenpox...(Pneumonia is a Hydrogen excess in the Liver...Think too much water...)

You can die from meningitis...(meningitis like Polio is also a fluorine excess in the Colon, a paralytic disease type-according to our chart which simplifies stuff down to just 11 organs...)

I got these ideas from an article that I was reading this morning about a girl, now a woman, a mother, who didn't get vaccinations as a child & knew others who didn't either...The above 4 possibilities(of maybe what could happen if you didn't get vaccinated) were actual people she knew...I am not going to cite the article or excerpt directly because this is a big topic for argument & I don't want to start an argument here...

Suffice it to say, there are good stories on both sides of the fence...To vaccinate or not to vaccinate that is the question...The bigger issue is that children don't get a say in much of all this...Maybe if children voiced their feelings more about all this, the dust might settle a bit...

Taking a cross up for another, I mean, speaking about someone else's life, even if they are a minor, is basically a violation of their privacy...I mean, how many children really want others to know if they are sick, got sick or not? Let them talk for themselves...

The hippy organic veggie lovechild who wrote how she now vaccinates her children, after a childhood of being ill all the time is a pervasive story...Told from the horse's mouth...Which is how I like to hear stuff!

The Basics:

How it works: Each organ contains two elements...A Minus Element & a Plus element...

These must live in balance...They are opposites...Disease is an imbalance...Figure out your own imbalance, then add its opposite to lower the excess...

Note:Elements are from the Periodic Table of Elements-these do not exist in the real world necessarily...On the linked pages I tell where to find those elements in real world items...

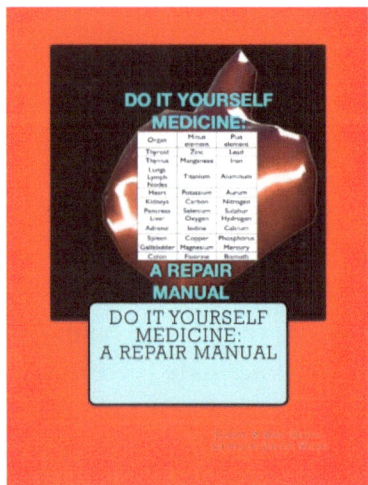

These are just a sample...Use this as a springboard for your own research...Be well! Sari Grove

Do it yourself medicine:A repair manual is built upon the foundations of the first book Grove Body Part Chart:A medical Arts Innovation...

This new work deals with more complicated problems, problems that may encompass several different imbalances at once...

It also looks more closely at the brain part to body part to elements connection...Which brain part controls what body part, & thusly which elements are involved...

It also takes a first look at sidedness...Once we know what brain part & what body part are involved & what elements, we can decide which side of the brain is affected, & also say which side of the brain contains predominantly which element...

The next picture looks at those examples...It also mentions how, if you follow the brain parts in order, as they attach to the body parts in order, how a spiral is formed by connecting each part...This confirms that our pattern is correct, as the spiral (called the Fibonacci spiral-think of a snail) is the building block of all things...

Getting hit on the nose makes the nose bigger because it swells up with Phosphorus, from the Spleen...

"Sidedness":stuff on the *left side of brain...

Brain
**appear on the RIGHT side of the body parts...*

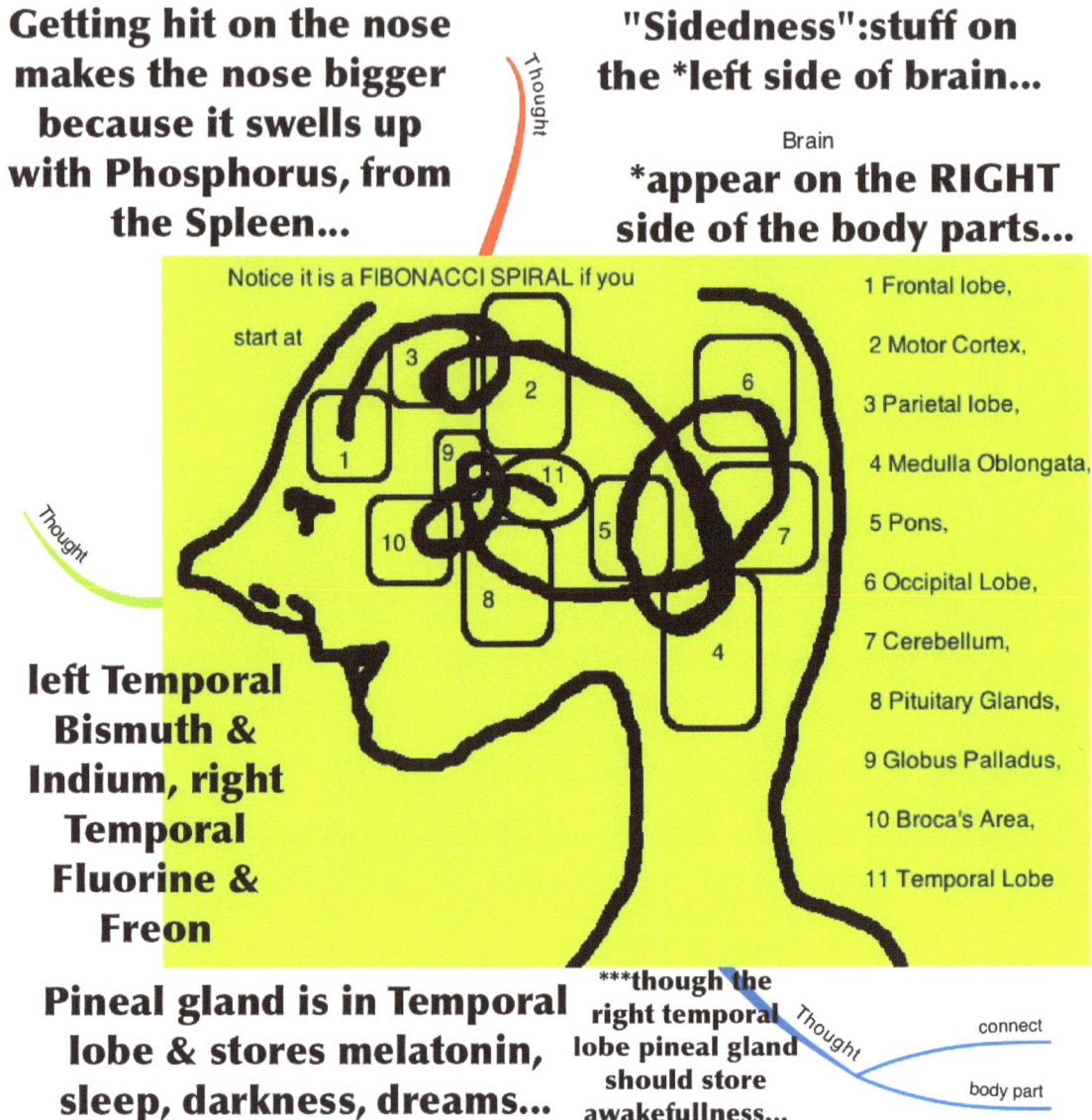

Notice it is a FIBONACCI SPIRAL if you start at

Thought

Thought

1 Frontal lobe,

2 Motor Cortex,

3 Parietal lobe,

4 Medulla Oblongata,

5 Pons,

6 Occipital Lobe,

7 Cerebellum,

8 Pituitary Glands,

9 Globus Palladus,

10 Broca's Area,

11 Temporal Lobe

left Temporal Bismuth & Indium, right Temporal Fluorine & Freon

Pineal gland is in Temporal lobe & stores melatonin, sleep, darkness, dreams...

***though the right temporal lobe pineal gland should store awakefullness...

Thought

connect

body part

The picture above shows several ideas at once...First, if you get hit in the Nose, it affects the Globus Palladus in the brain (number 9), then it affects the Spleen, which contains both Phosphorus & Copper...The injury causes an EXCESS of Phosphorus, which is like mold, & over a very long period of time, can cause Parkinson's disease, which is an excess of Phosphorus that is now more systemic...Like a mold infestation...Thus, Parkinson's disease, Spleen damage, & getting hit in the nose, can all be treated with Copper things...Copper is found in Coffee...The better the coffee, the more copper is in it...(I drink Jamaican Blue Mountain coffee pressed through a Bodum French Press)...(drink with a Hot Straw to keep my teeth whiter)....

The second thing the picture speaks to is the tendency for things on the LEFT side of the brain to be PLUS elements...Things on the RIGHT side of the brain tend to be MINUS elements...So, looking at the Temporal lobe, you might find Bismuth(& Indium is similar but stronger) on the Left side of the temporal lobe...You'd find its opposite & Minus element, Fluorine, on the RIGHT side of the brain...Which means that on the RIGHT side of the BODY, you'd find PLUS dominant things-because the brain cross switches to the body...Cross switches means what exists on the right brain acts out on the LEFT body, & vice versa...

The third thing the picture shows is that as you progress from the first brain part, the Frontal lobe, all the way down the list of brain parts that correspond to the way the BODY parts flow, that you get a Fibonacci spiral...The spiral is the building block, well, building spiral of everything...Think of a snail to understand the spiral...The strongest structures are built on a spiral...The planets...Your thoughts travel along curved lines...

Each Organ has 2 Opposing Elements...(Minus & Plus)

Organ	Minus Element	Plus Element
Thyroid	Zinc	Lead
Thymus	Manganese	Iron
Lungs & Lymph Nodes	Titanium	Aluminum
Heart	Potassium	Aurum
Kidneys	Carbon	Nitrogen
Pancreas	Selenium	Sulphur
Liver	Oxygen	Hydrogen
Adrenal Gland	Iodine	Calcium
Spleen	Copper	Phosphorus
Gallbladder	Magnesium	Mercury
Colon	Fluorine	Bismuth

This is the chart...Each organ contains a Minus element & a Plus element...Minus elements are cleansers they detox, Plus elements are nutrifiers, give nutrition...Adding one will lower the other...For example, adding Manganese will lower your Iron levels, in the Thymus...(if you have Lice for instance, you want to LOWER iron...Black walnut hull powder is a manganese that does this fast)...Most health problems are imbalance problems...Too much of one thing, or not enough of another...

My newer theory about sidedness is basically, that in the brain, the left side of the brain is PLUS element dominant...Which means the RIGHT side of the body is PLUS element dominant...

So when you look at my brain part to body part connections, add the idea that for that brain part, the left side of the brain will contain the Plus element of the body part that it connects to...

For example, if you destroy the left side of the frontal lobe, which should contain the Plus element which is LEAD, then you will be right frontal brain dominant, & your ZINC side will take over...Zinc dominance shows up as Bipolar disorder...So you would know that if you had removed the left frontal lobe you need to supplement with Lead things like carrot juice(Vitamin A is a Lead thing)...

Just to clarify very specifically:DAMAGE to an Organ results in a Plus element excess...REMOVAL of an Organ results in a Minus element excess....For example, damage to the Spleen causes Phosphorus excess, a Plus element...Removing the Gallbladder causes a Minus element excess of Magnesium excess....So removing an organ & damage to an organ give entirely OPPOSITE results....

The sidedness theory should help people with specific side brain damage...To know what element has been lost & what to replenish with...

Homeostasis just means the state of the body parts being all in the right place at the right time with the right amounts of everything inside...The body & the brain tend towards homeostasis, meaning it is a self-cleaning oven...It self-balances...Which means that sometimes if you just leave something alone, it will get better...Part of the Hippocratic oath for doctors...Physicians...Also something your dad might tell you...

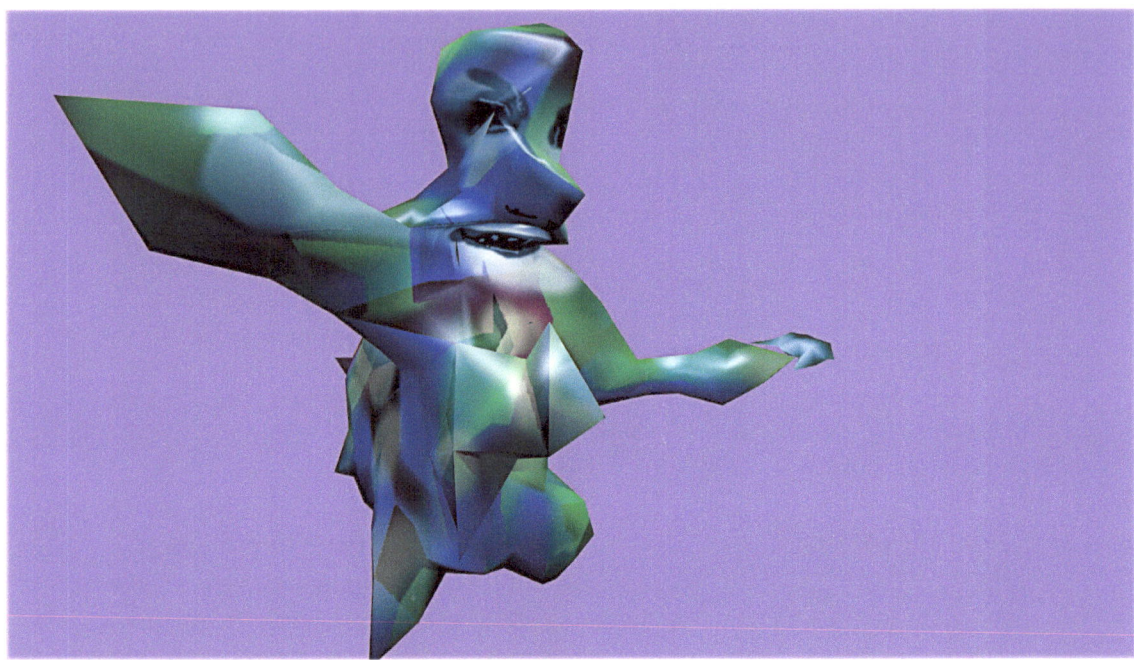

1.

2. Some people use the Holy Bible as a health guide...Some people follow the latest cultural habits to get well, like smoking cigarettes to get Zinc in low sunshine lands...Some people use exercise like QiGong, or hold down 2 jobs to get more exercise...Some people move to places like France where the food is better quality & fast foods are shunned...Decide what kind of person you are, then choose your regimen based on your tastes, your location, the culture of where you live, the climate, or your favorite foods...Sometimes instinct or looking back at what you have already done gives hints as to what kind of person or animal you are...Don't do something that irks you...

3. "To thine own self be true", Shakespeare wrote...

4. Someone's wise daughter once explained that if you were attracted to a certain rock, a mineral, it might be that it is good for you...(Earth Rocks is in Toronto now at Bathurst & Bloor...)

Before we look at the Chart,let's continue to look at some overarching principles, in particular, those that are affecting people right now...Today...

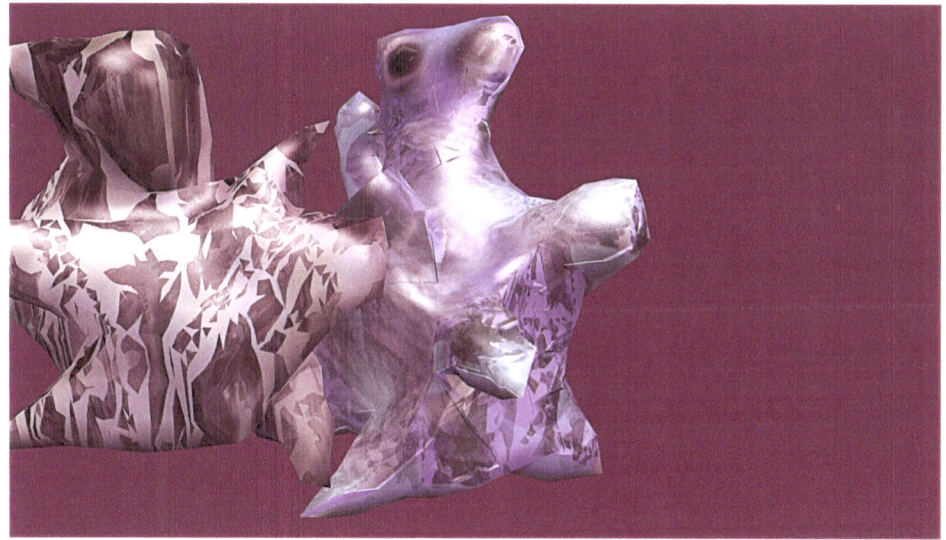

Do it yourself medicine: a repair manual
Grove Body Part Chart

each organ has two opposite elements

Organ	Minus element	Plus element
Thyroid	Zinc	Lead
Thymus	Manganese	Iron
Lungs Lymph Nodes	Titanium	Aluminum
Heart	Potassium	Aurum
Kidneys	Carbon	Nitrogen
Pancreas	Selenium	Sulphur
Liver	Oxygen	Hydrogen
Adrenal	Iodine	Calcium
Spleen	Copper	Phosphorus
Gallbladder	Magnesium	Mercury
Colon	Fluorine	Bismuth

Frontal Lobe

Motor Cortex

Pons

globus palladus

temporal lobe

Parietal Lobe

medulla oblongata

occipital lobe

cerebellum

pituitary gland

Broca's area

Each stem on the picture is connected specifically to the organ & 2 elements it interacts with...For example, Broca's area at the bottom left hand stem connects to the Gallbladder which contains both Magnesium & Mercury...assume during an imbalance effect that all of those systems may be involved, including the speech lips & mouth which also are involved with Broca's area & so on(Later I have pictures showing more specifics of what things the brain parts do)...

Since Broca's area & Wernicke's area are both ruled by the Temporal Lobe which rules the Gallbladder-though Broca's produces speech while Wernicke's works with listening & understanding speech, AND, Broca's sits towards the front, & Wernicke's towards the back, of the head, of the brain, THEN, one MIGHT POSIT, that, things towards the front of the brain/head are more concerned with outward producing things, while things towards the back of the head/brain, are concerned with INNER thoughts, logic, processing information things...In skiing, men fall forward & women fall back...Center of Gravity gender difference...So men like giant slalom & women like moguls...Slalom leans forward, Moguls lean back to bend...So do women have more brain activity in the BACK of the head & men more in the front? (The bias in male physician history is that frontal activity is for smarter people, but that's just because more men were physicians back then & they were just describing a male tendency...Hence our new terminology of Emotional Intelligence- a defense of the back headed thought dominant female perhaps?)

Within the Temporal lobe, which connects to the Colon with Bismuth & Fluorine inside, there is the Pineal gland which handles light & dark or sleep & awake, whilst in the same temporal Lobe, Wernicke's area handles understanding (listening as opposed to speaking), with the left side of Wernicke's being the Plus element side, let's say the Bismuth side, since Bismuth is our Plus for the Colon, & those thoughts are the Dominant type thoughts that are more commonly understood, like the sky is blue or water is wet...The right side, or Minus side of Wernicke's area handles thoughts & understanding that are non-dominant, like the sky is orange at sunset, or Perrier water is bubbly...Understanding & ears are affected in the Colon, as is balance...The type of thoughts you are having, if you are feeling odd or unwell, might indicate which imbalance you have...Are your thoughts all abstract? Perhaps you have a Fluorine excess, because Fluorine lives on the right side of Wernicke's in the temporal lobe, & handles abstract thoughts... Are your thoughts mundane, cliche, stereotypical, common? Perhaps you have a Bismuth excess? Are you also constipated? Bismuth constipates in excess, that might confirm that direction...

Next big thought:

Subject: Ca+ Plus element=Cancer in that Organ
Date: Tue, 07 Jan 2014 04:04:34 -0500

Calcium plus mercury= gallstones

Ca+Uric acid Nitrogen=kidney stones

Ca+Iron=Leukemia Blood thymus involvement

Ca+Lead in Thyroid Gland=Bone Cancer

Ca+The Plus Element in any organ =Cancer in that Organ

Ok, so the above phrases are formulas...Cancer is calcium excess in the Adrenal Gland, usually today caused by somehow getting a birth control drug into your system(from your mom, from your spouse, from contact, from taking them, from the location of your water supply, etc.)... Now that Calcium excess ends up in various places in your body... It tends to stick where there is another excess or predisposition of a PLus element...Say you are Irish or just naturally high in Iron in the Thymus which makes blood...The calcium floats around & settles in your Thymus, sticking to the iron there...Now your Bloodmaking is affected...That is cancer of the blood...Just Calcium + Iron...They call that Leukemia... Ok, so now you get the formula... The Thyroid gland makes bone...Calcium added to a high Lead level there makes...What? Bone Cancer...Because the Thyroid makes bone...

How does Calcium(birth control pills) get into the Breasts? Well birth control pills contain inactive ingredients, like maybe gelatin for example as a binder...What exactly is gelatin? Well, let's look at suet, that fatty stuff with birdseed in it you give to birds in winter to keep them warm...The fat part is beef tallow...Tallow is very high in cholesterol...Cholesterol is an Aluminum element on our chart...Aluminum lives in the Lungs & Lymph Nodes on our chart...The breasts sit on top of the Lungs & Lymph Nodes...So if you eat a calcium pill(birth control pill) that has a gelatin coating(Aluminum element), then that pill might want to migrate to your Lung & Lymph node system...Maybe in the fatty part where Aluminum levels are highest...Boom...They get stuck there & now you have a lump of birth control pills stuck in your boob...Which is why you may need a multi-pronged attack to get rid of Cancers(Calciums) that show up outside the Adrenal Gland...Like in your boobs(sorry, my words), which are part of the Lungs system, to offset or remove extra Aluminum you need a Titanium...Also you need an Iodine to remove the main problem the Cancer, Calcium...So depending on where that calcium lump shows up in your body, also try to lower the PLUS element specifically in that ORGAN...

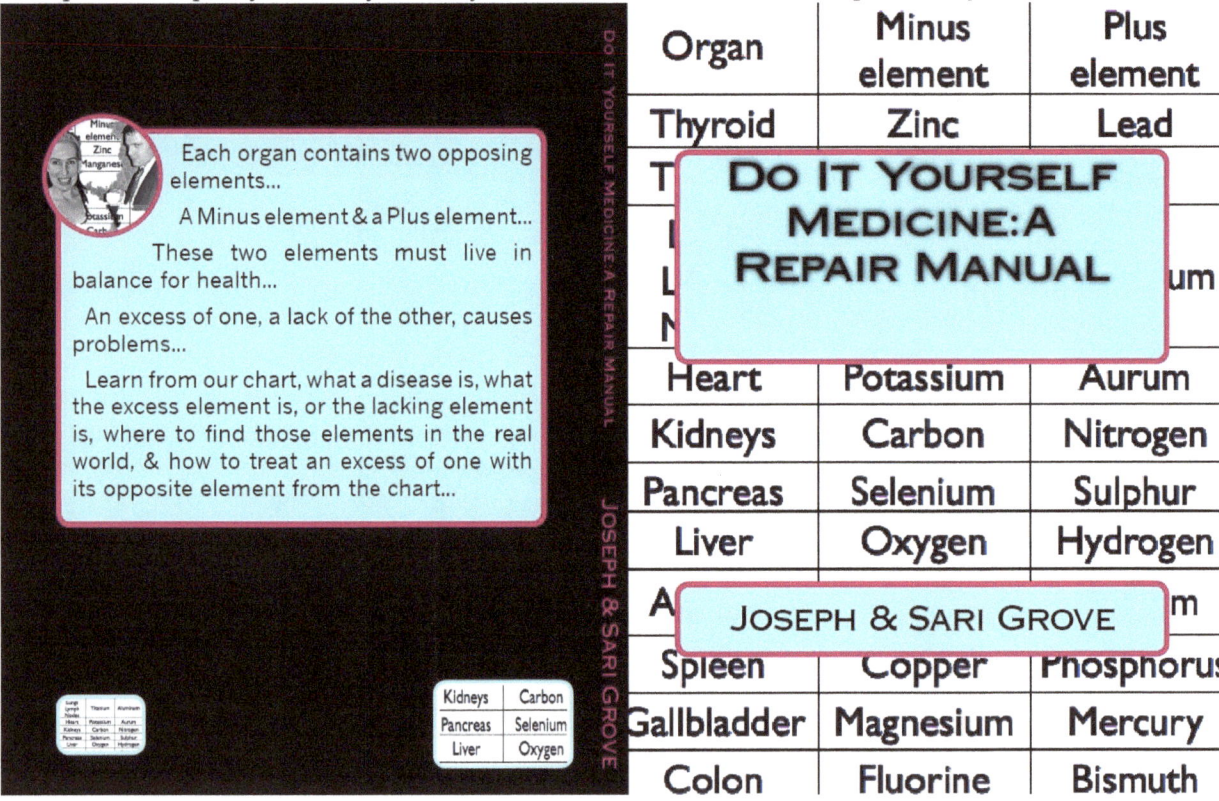

Organ	Minus element	Plus element
Thyroid	Zinc	Lead
		um
Heart	Potassium	Aurum
Kidneys	Carbon	Nitrogen
Pancreas	Selenium	Sulphur
Liver	Oxygen	Hydrogen
A		m
Spleen	Copper	Phosphorus
Gallbladder	Magnesium	Mercury
Colon	Fluorine	Bismuth

Each organ contains two opposing elements...

A Minus element & a Plus element...

These two elements must live in balance for health...

An excess of one, a lack of the other, causes problems...

Learn from our chart, what a disease is, what the excess element is, or the lacking element is, where to find those elements in the real world, & how to treat an excess of one with its opposite element from the chart...

DO IT YOURSELF MEDICINE:A REPAIR MANUAL

JOSEPH & SARI GROVE

"When I'm working on a problem, I never think about beauty. I think only how to solve the problem. But when I have finished, if the solution is not beautiful, I know it is wrong."
-- R. Buckminster Fuller

(This is my own Amazon review on Amazon of this book...Heh!...)
First I should state, I am the author! Yes...I am Sari Grove(ok, one of the authors)...But my opinion still counts don't you think?
So...

The chart, the Grove Body Part Chart, which is the basis for this book & the previous one (Grove Body Part Chart:A medical Arts innovation), is really neat...neat? Well, it sorts through the body down to 11 organs & then shows the 2 elements in each of those organs that must live in balance as opposites in order to maintain health...

That chart can simplify many people's understanding of their own health...With so many words, long long words, & complicated explanations in medicine, it is really refreshing to get something that makes it all so much simpler...

Once you"get" the Chart idea, then you can sail along to whatever it is you are seeking...

Sections are devoted to each body part, which excess of what element is what disease or imbalance, & where to find those elements(from the Periodic Table of Elements) in the real world...

As a paperback, this book is a handy reference guide that pretty much anyone can use...

You can find out what the imbalance is of whatever disease you have been diagnosed with, & maybe you could even find its opposite element in the real world, to aid in your own treatment...

Some of those neat ideas include: Say you have scleroderma...Find that in the Lead excess section in the Thyroid gland...Find its opposite element on the Chart...Ah, Zinc...Find out where Zinc is found in the real world...Ah, sunshine contains Zinc...Schedule a trip to somewhere sunny or buy yourself a great bikini & some coconut oil & start suntanning! You are now one step closer to health...Did you know that in fact phototherapy is the number one treatment for Scleroderma? With this book, you get answers right away...Not to replace your traditional medical choices, but to make yourself more educated...It is YOUR body isn't it?

See why Alzheimer's disease is NOT CAUSED by Aluminum...See how the common cold & depression are worsened with alcohol & even water, all Hydrogens! (Why people are told to drink plenty of fluids when they have a cold is just so WRONG)...

There are pictures throughout the book, mostly just to liven up the reading...But the pictures that are really worthwhile are the ones of the brain part to body part connection...Sure people have mapped the brain before, but they have hedged their bets with a huge amount of yeses & nos...Boiling it all down to this brain part connects to this body part is a bold move...Not only that, Sari(me) attempts to posit a theory about sidedness...That the left side of the brain parts are PLus element dominant, as are the right side of the body parts...This is a bold move forward in the field of neurology...

The author(me again) is the daughter of a neuro-ophthalmological surgeon & professor to medical students...The author's husband & co-author(Joseph Grove) is grandson to an Oxford educated Physician who also served in the military prior to getting his Rhodes scholarship...So these two people sort of have a knack for understanding medical concepts, & take them further, into the art of healing...In fact, both of these people call themselves artists...Because only with experience in the arts, with creativity & innovation, can anyone break free from accepted principles & pioneer new ideas...

Ok...Have I gone too far? It's a good book...You will probably want a hard copy(a paper version) to keep handy in your home, office, boat or wherever...or to gift to a friend...It is pricier because of all the colour images, but honestly it would be boring without the pictures...Art is so integral to health, why take the art out of the book just to make it cheaper?

Anyways, I hope I got the ball rolling, review-wise...

If anyone has already read the book, & it has helped them in any way, please mention that in a review here...I feel the bare no review look is so spare looking...Let's warm this place up! Sari

p.s.If anyone has any problems with anything in the book, please write to me & I can upload a revision...(Yes, I can edit out big mistakes if necessary!)
*end of review... grove@sent.com to write me directly...

What follows:

What follows is the Chart in order from top of the body to the bottom, with then a more detailed look at each body part later on...Within the detailed look is the brain part to body part connection sketches...Again, for sidedness, I am saying that the left side of the brain is Plus element dominant, & the right side of the body is Plus element dominant...& VICE VERSA for the other side of the brain & body...So the RIGHT side of the brain should be MINUS element dominant, & the LEFT side of the body should also be MINUS element dominant...

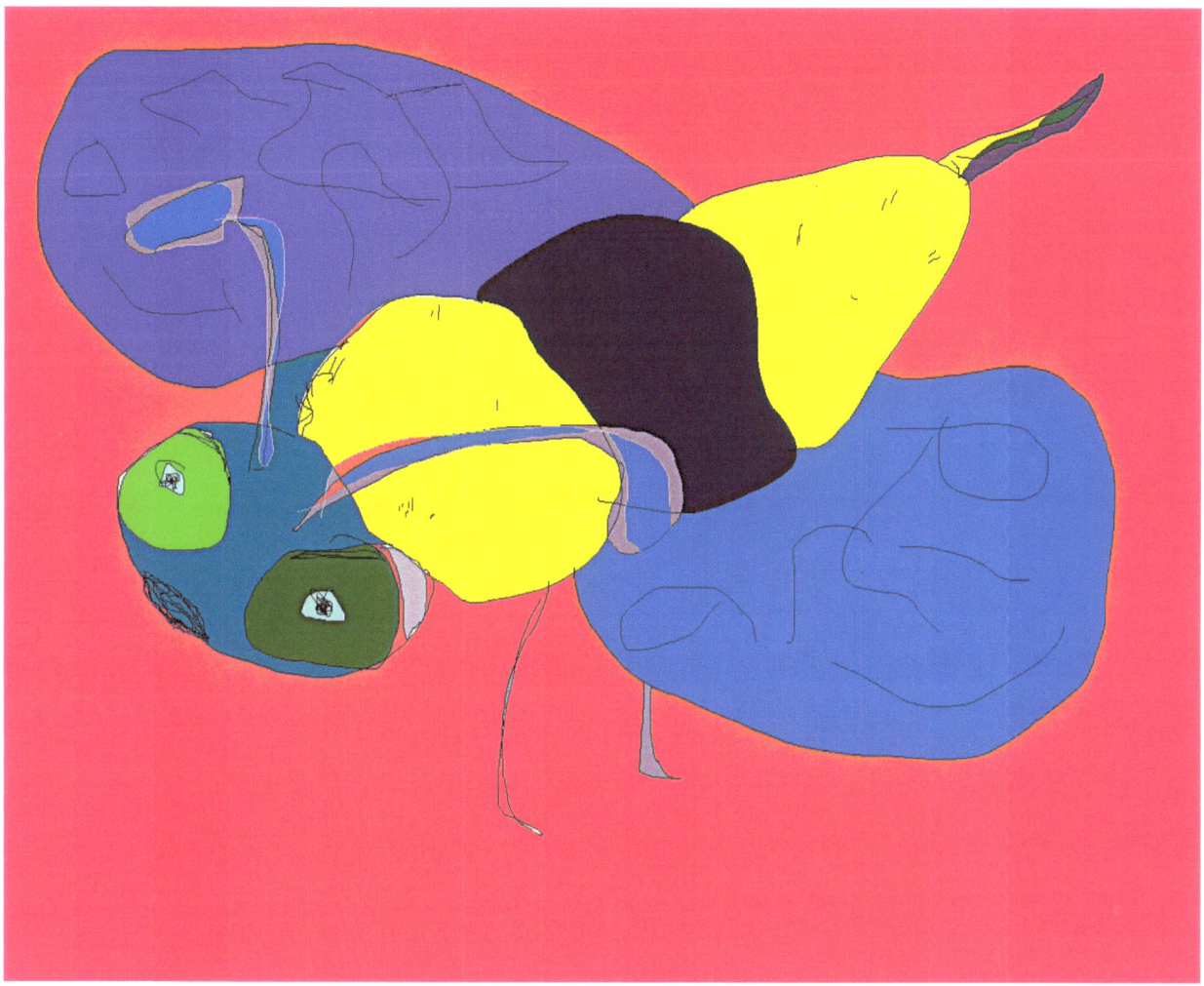

"Out beyond ideas of wrong doing and right doing, there is a field; I'll meet you there."
from a Rumi poem

1)Thyroid = Zinc + Lead

5. Bipolar Thalidomide Agent Orange Leprosy Frontal Lobe degradation of BONES , **LEFT** side of FRONTAL lobe removal associated with bipolar-the left side contains the Lead so removal there causes excess Zinc which is on the right frontal lobe, - artists who are lefties have right frontal brain dominance which is the ZINC side so they are more impulsive types-they have more Zinc-*remember right frontal zinc brain controls left side of body like the hand!(Zinc excess)

6.

7. (Lead excess)Multiple Sclerosis, Parasites ,Roundworms, Pinworms, Lice, Malaria, Lupus, Aspergillosis, Scleroderma(Lead excess)

8.

9.

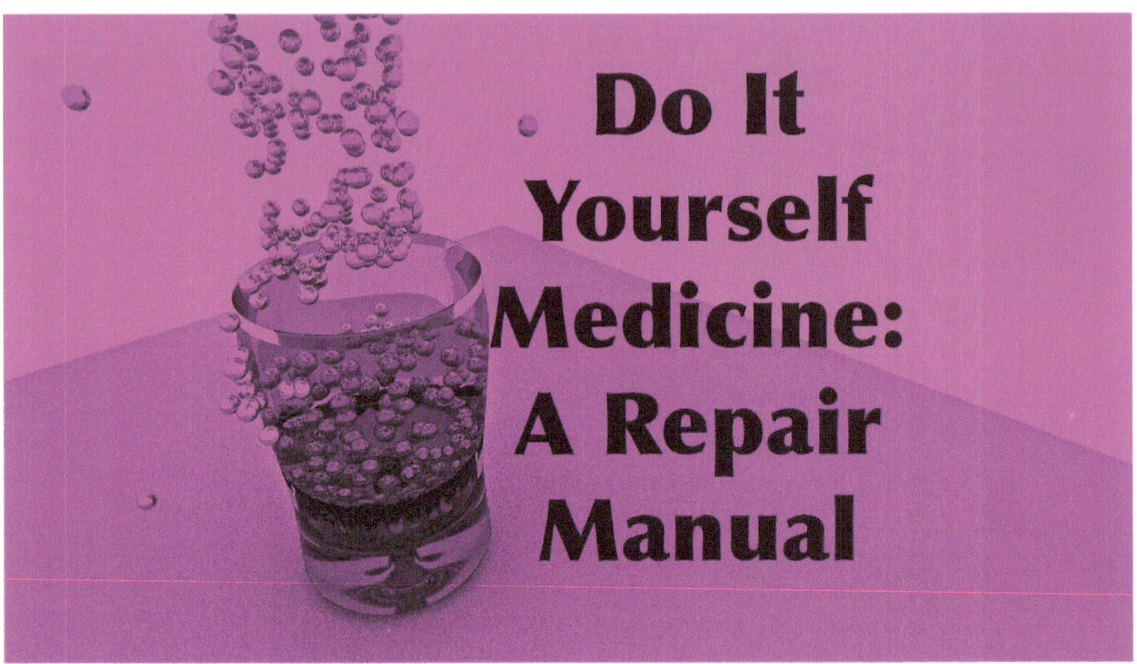

2)Thymus = Manganese + Iron

10. PTSD Post traumatic Stress Disorder Iron Anemia BLOOD , Reynaud's syndrome or Reynaud's phenomenon-fingers & toes that turn blue or white when cold & back to red when warm(Manganese excess)

11.

12.

13. (Iron excess)Hemachromatosis Myasthenia Gravis Lice infestation(Iron excess)

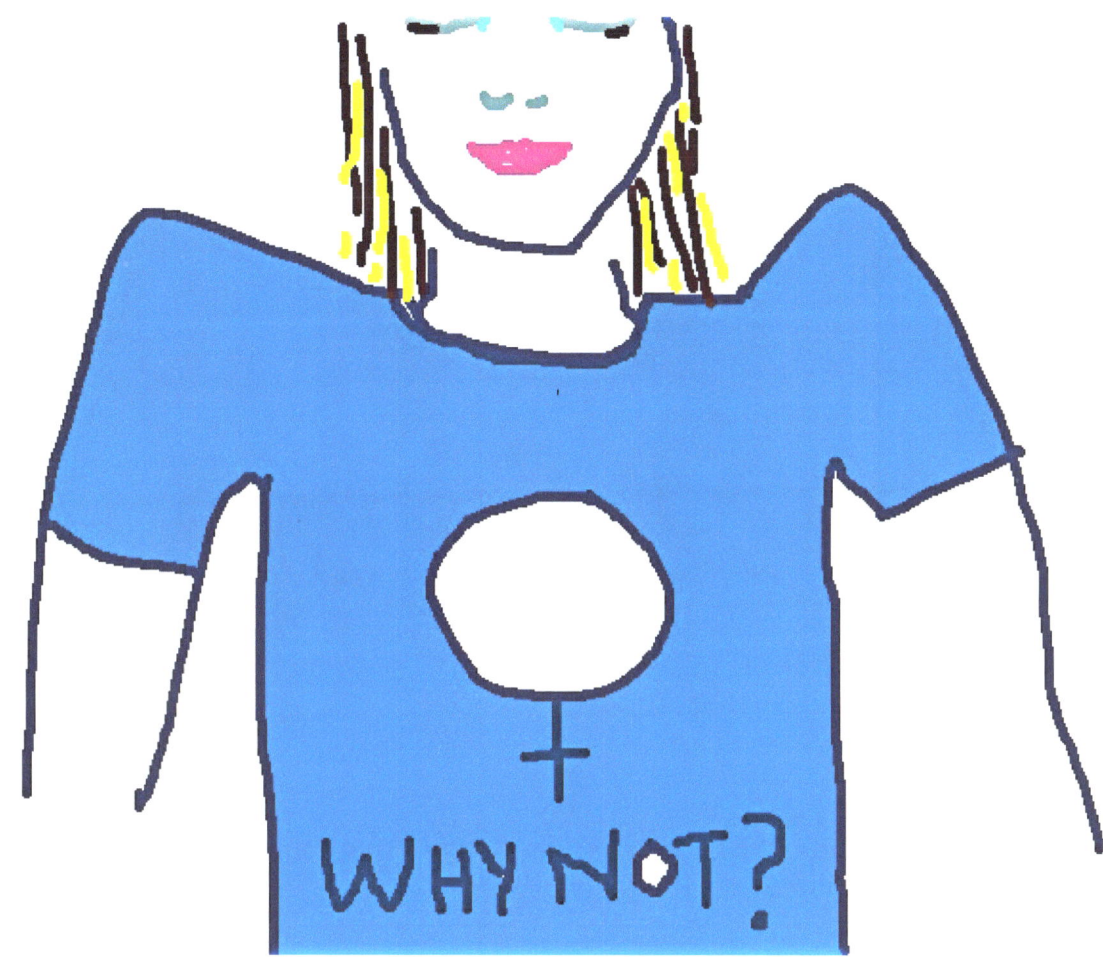

"You see things; and you say, 'Why?' But I dream things that never were; and I say, "Why not?"
George Bernard Shaw

14. 3)Lungs Lymph Nodes = Titanium + Aluminum

15. Alzheimer's Disease Schizophrenia Cerebral Palsy Anxiety & OCD Haemophilia
     Hyperhidrosis/Sweatyness MUSCLES, clang and jang titanium-"clang & jang"
     syndrome means you are rhyming words accidentally, when you speak-it is a sign of
     possible schizophrenia which is a Titanium excess(Titanium excess)

16.

17. (Aluminum excess)Asthma Tuberculosis Pulmonary Hypertension Consumption Cystic
     Fibrosis Trouble Breathing(Aluminum excess)

18.

19.

20.

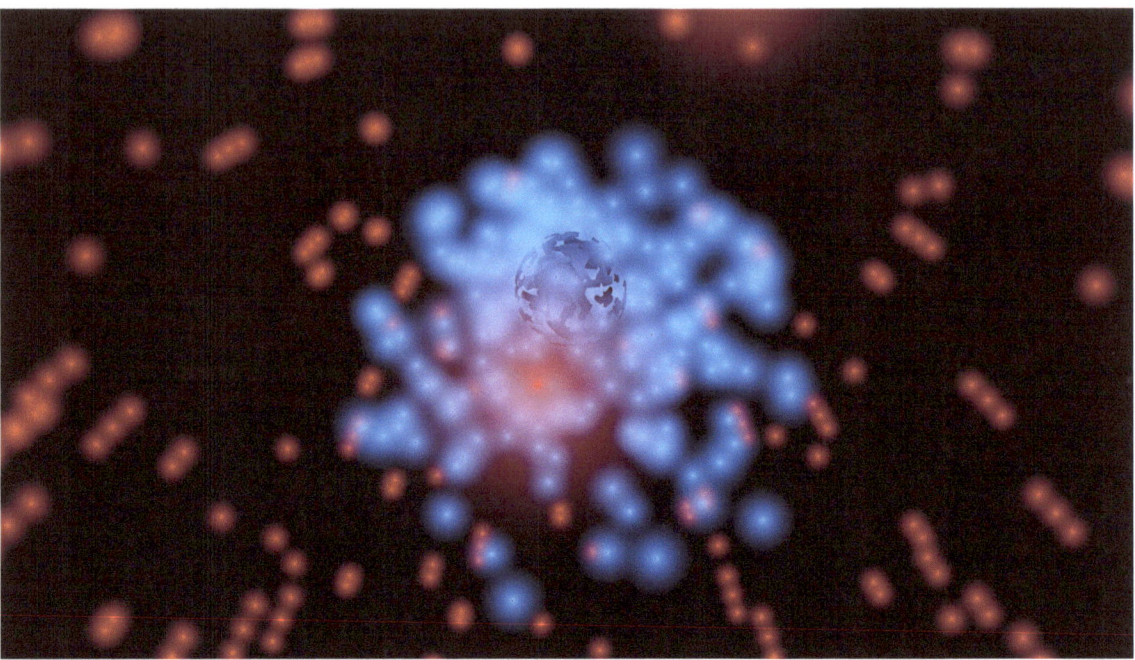

4)Heart = Potassium + Aurum

21. HCM HypertrophicCardioMyopathy (weak but enlarged heart distended low blood pressure) Concussion Vasovagal Attack Epileptic seizures also have a Low Taurine High Potassium component though Epilepsy is primarily a Fluorine excess syndrome-see Colon SEALS & VALVES(Potassium excess)

22.

23. (Aurum, Gold excess)Clogged heart (small size but congested high blood pressure) (Aurum excess)

24.

25.

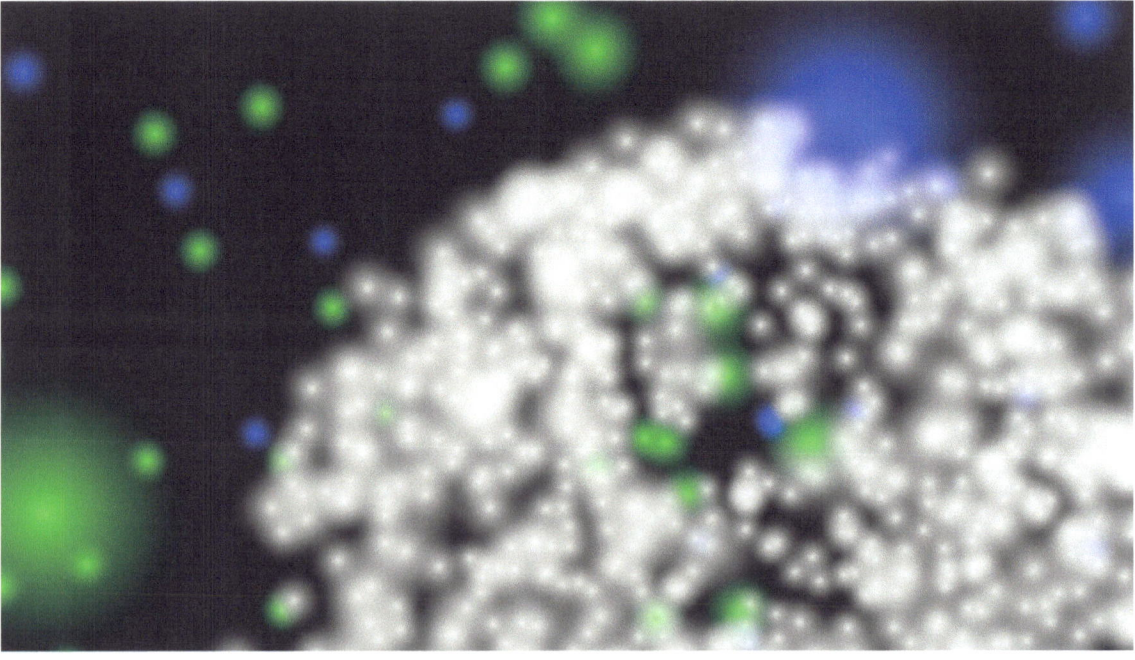

5)Kidneys = Carbon + Nitrogen

26. Down's Syndrome NEURONS & NERVES & RENAL TUBES *Living near to a highway may/causes Carbon excess-Misunderstanding people in conversation might be the first sign the Carbon from the cars is affecting your intelligence(Carbon Excess)
27.
28. (Nitrogen excess)Kidney blockages failures Celiac & any other gluten problems (Nitrogen excess)
29. Kidney Failure Blockages Aggression/Hateful nature
30. Nitrogen excess can also trigger stroke
31. I am putting GOUT here also as a Nitrogen excess...(see further along, for my reasons, in the Kidneys section)...
32.

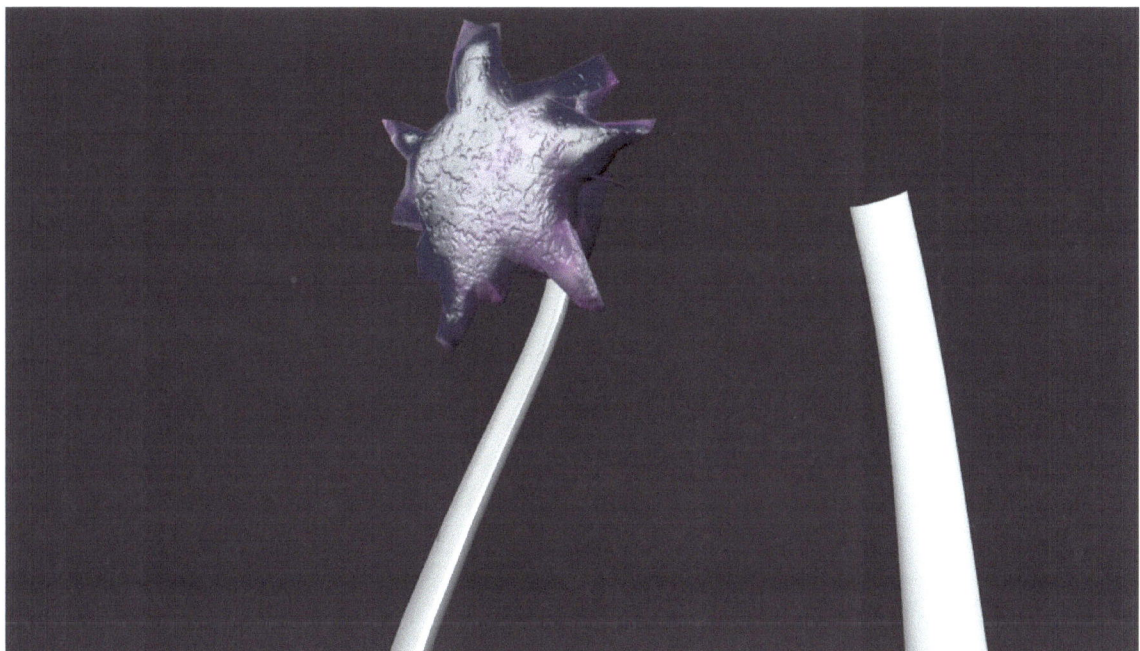

6)Pancreas = Selenium + Sulphur

33.
34. (Sulphur excess)Diabetes Herpes Dandruff Pimples Rotten teeth & gums(Sulphur excess-sulphur is in sugar)Blindness can occur with diabetes sugars excess Macular Degeneration of the eye diabetes related, Glaucoma, diabetic retinopathy, EYES, Infections anywhere...Also Sulphur excess is characteristic of Measles Rubella & Chicken Pox...
35.
36. (Selenium excess): Bad breath(garlicky), low blood sugar hypoglycemia, faint, dizzy
37.
38.

 7)Liver = Oxygen + Hydrogen
39. Dehydration dry mouth (Oxygen Excess)
40.

41. (Hydrogen excess)Common Cold Chronic Fatigue Syndrome Chronic Severe Depression Suicidal ME Myalgic Encephalomyelitis Hepatitis B Hydrocephalic water on the brain brain swollen Cirrhosis Migraine HYDRATION Pneumonia (Hydrogen Excess)

42.

43.

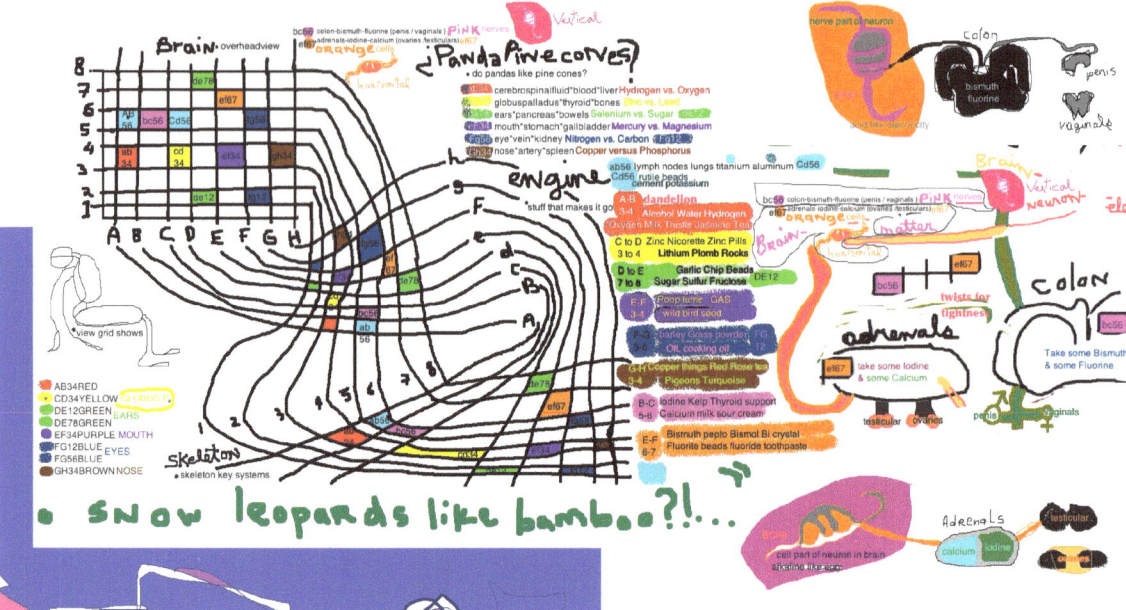

9)Adrenal Gland = Iodine + Calcium

44. Grave's disease Addison's disease(Iodine excess)

45.

46. (Calcium excess)Cancer Obesity(female) Underweight(male)Lack of love feelings Endometriosis Breast cancer Ovarian Cancer Prostate Cancer Lung Cancer STRENGTH MILK, Overbreeding of the Mother leading to Gender Dysphoria in the Offspring AIDS Skin Cancer Damaged adrenal gland with calcium excess due to birth control drugs/progesterones/calciums, damaged adrenal gland due to overbreeding of the mother, Celibacy, Celibate behaviours due to Vitex agnus castus/a calcium herbal, the monk's salt...(Calcium excess)

47. (***The picture below mentions Aragonite sand, which is a Calcium Carbonate sand which I use to make homemade marble & also to make my concrete recipes stickier...Aragonite sand, as a calcium & carbon based sand, is safer for reptiles & fish & waterbirds...I was designing a 5 sided nest for Trumpeter swans, to be filled with Aragonite sand, & designated just for them, at the beach area of Bluffer's Park in Toronto...Beach real estate needs to be reserved, so that our native Trumpeter Swans can have some beach area to rest on, that cannot be disturbed by people & their children & their dogs...Sometimes, these 5 sided nests, need to be enclosed with an opening to the water, to provide further protection from stray predators...

48.

Nest swan
Sand shape

2.5 ft
wood. bag of

dishes & leaves

grass?
moss rock
wild bird seed

5 feet

seaweed kelp

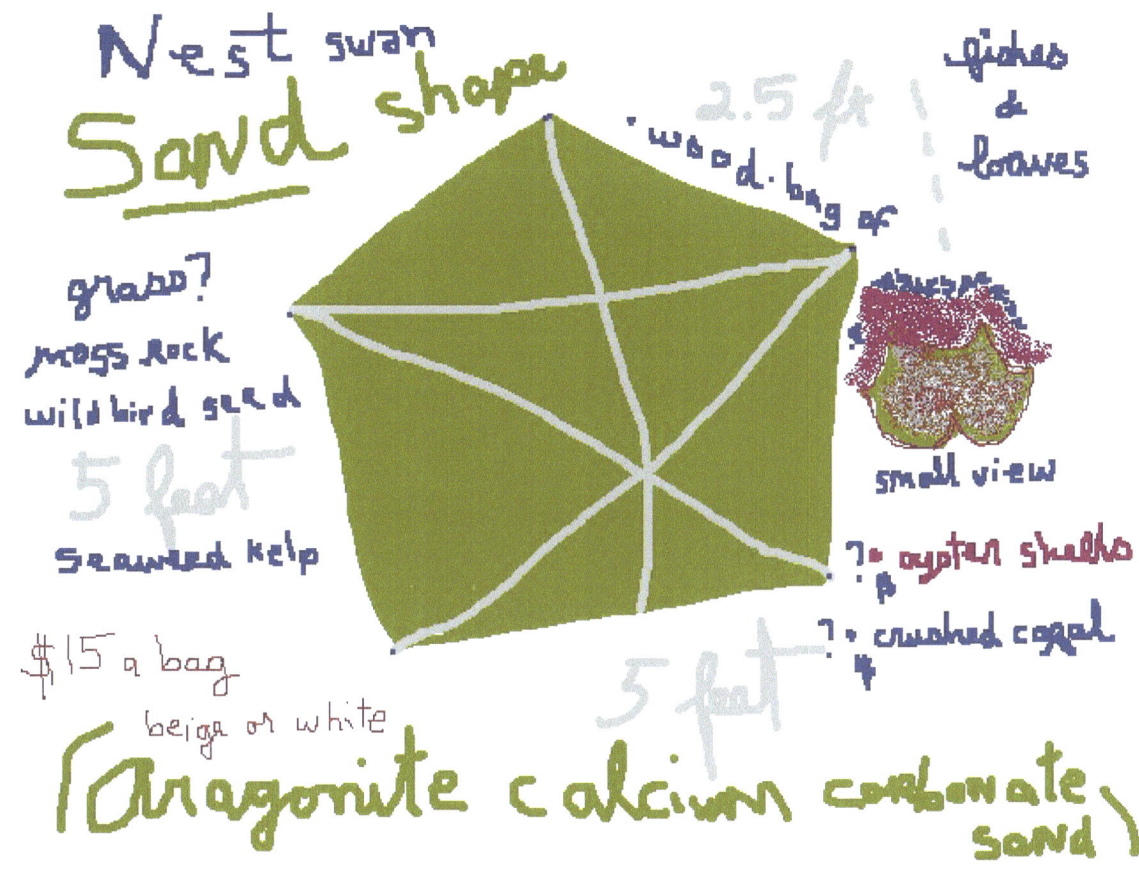

small view

?. oyster shells

?. crushed coral

$15 a bag

beige or white

5 feet

(aragonite calcium carbonate sand)

49.

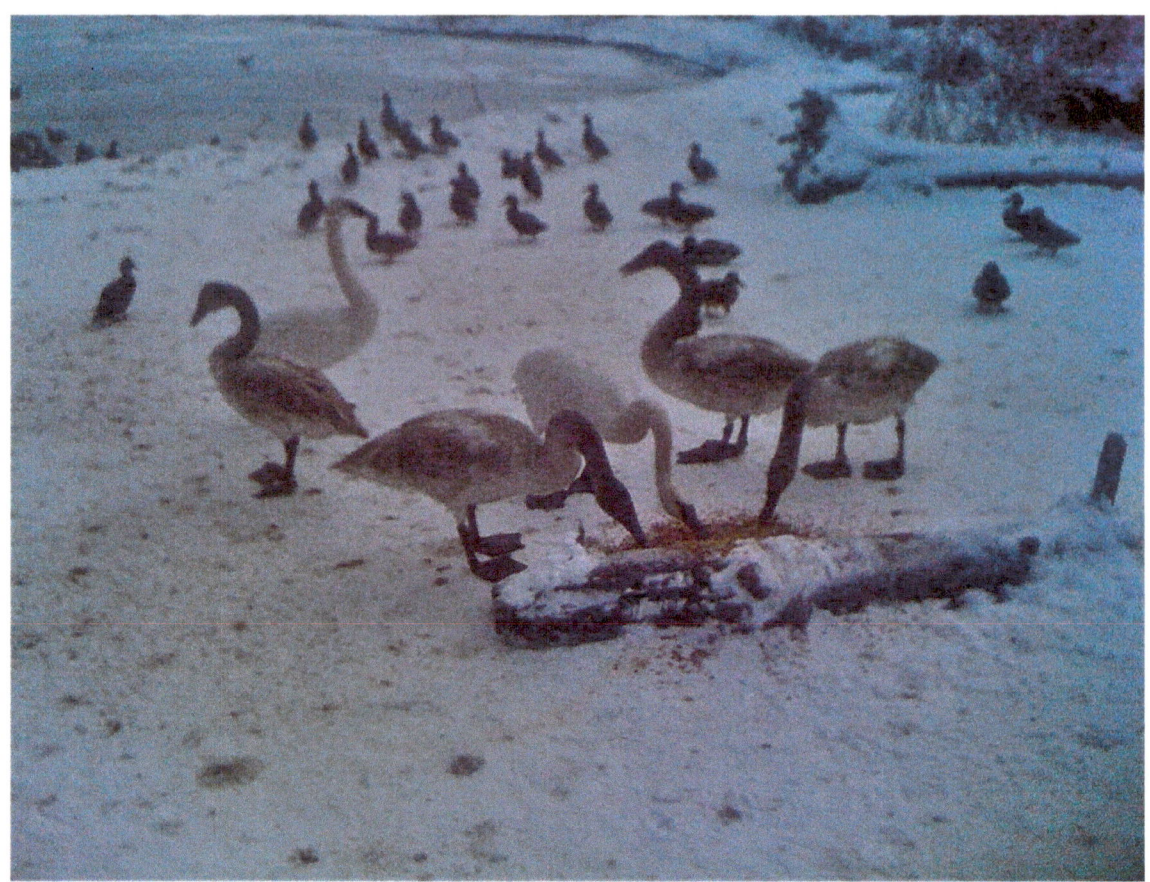

(6 month old Trumpeter Swan cygnets in the snow & ice at Bluffer's Park Dec. 28, 2013)

50.

51. 8)Spleen = Copper + Phosphorus

52. Rushing speeding Acid reflux(Copper excess)

53.

54. (Phosphorus excess)Parkinson's disease Tremor Lack of sexual desire feeling Salmonella NOSE(Phosphorus excess)

55.

56.

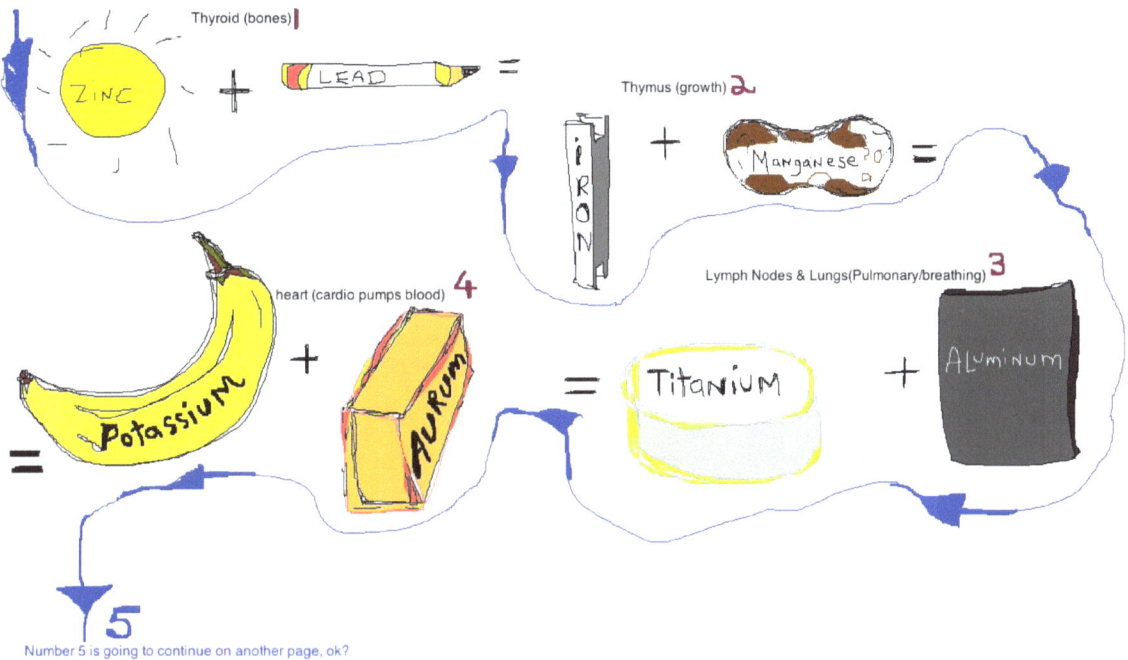

10)Gallbladder = Magnesium + Mercury

57. Arthritis Joint degeneration knee hip jaw elbow shoulder ankle cartilage loss Still's disease Meningitis mean rude personality Need for hip replacement Fibromyalgia, MOUTH TENDONS CARTILAGE Poohing too much diarrhea(can also be other elements too so check-but magnesium is a strong laxative for sure!)

58.

59.

60. (Mercury excess)Gallstones ADHD ADD Asperger's Violent Violence Lyme Disease *Living near to a sewage treatment plant raises Mercury levels-early signs are violent/ violence reactions to small things Also, Creutzfeldt-Jakob-also known as BSE Bovine Spongiform Encephalophy or Mad Cow disease (Mercury excess)

61.

62.

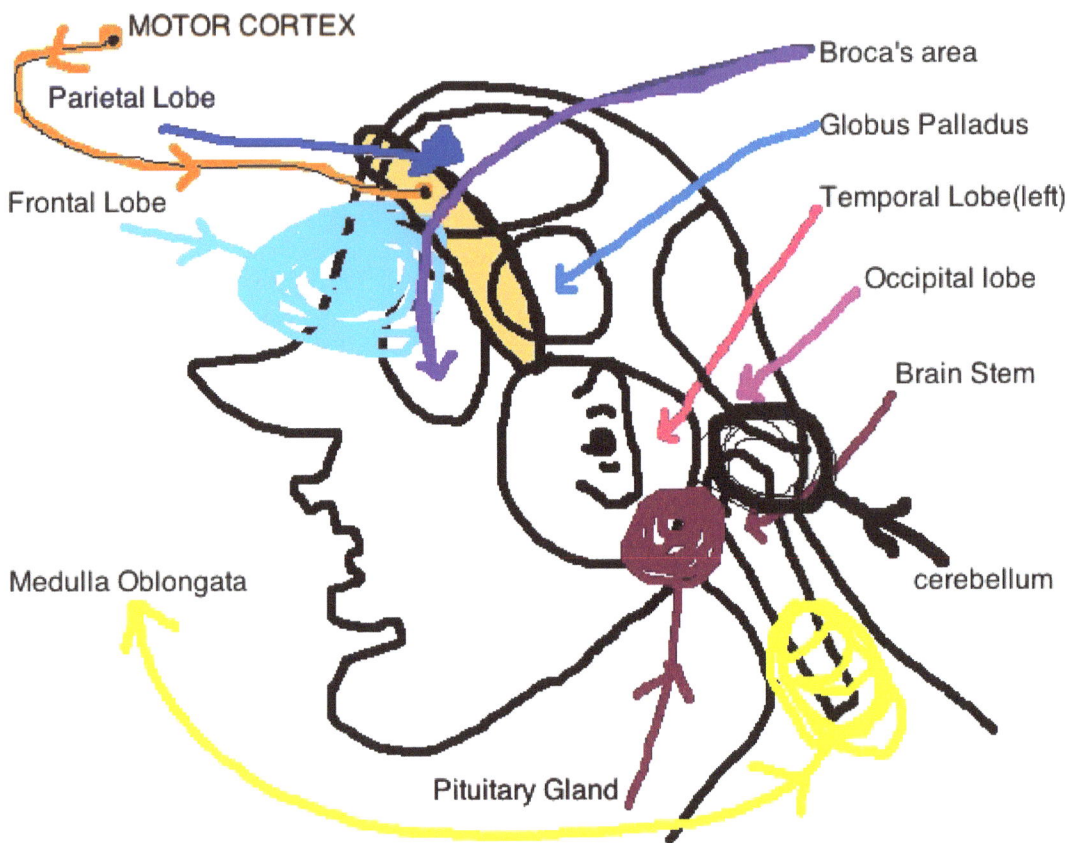

11)Colon= Fluorine + Bismuth

63. (Fluorine excess)ALS Amyolotrophic Lateral Sclerosis Lou Gehrig's disease Crohn's disease Epilepsy Seizures the orphan illness Fabry(with hearing loss)Gulf War syndrome Double Aortic Arch Vascular Ring Cholera Typhus Diarrhea Angelman's Syndrome Huntington's disease Guillain-Barre Syndrome Tetanus Syringomyelia EARS(Fluorine excess)

64.

1.   On each Page of this blog(book) I have also added how that organ connects to what place in the brain & what functions, as well as elements that feed that part of the brain & that body part...Knowing the elements can help you decide course of treatment if there is an imbalance...I also drew all the pictures using Mac's free Paint program! Sari Grove Thanksgiving in Canada Monday October 14, 2013

65.

READ OUR BOOK! See it below, embedded as a PDF(only online)! Tell Sari what you think at grove@sent.com

66. Grove Body Part Chart:A Medical Arts Innovation(each organ contains 2 opposing elements) by GroveCanada:Joseph & Sari Grove

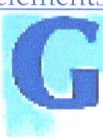

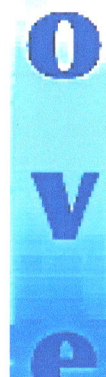
(OUR FIRST BOOK IS AVAILABLE FOR FREE ON OUR BLOG AS A PDF)...

1.   scribd (is where you can read our two books digitally...We are GroveCanada on http://www.Scribd.com Read Grove Body Part Chart:A Medical Arts Innovation, first...then this book after...Do it Yourself Medicine:A Repair Manual...

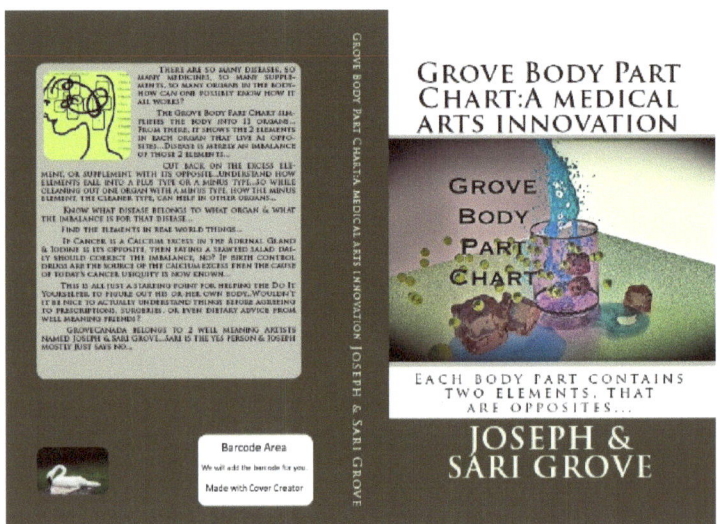

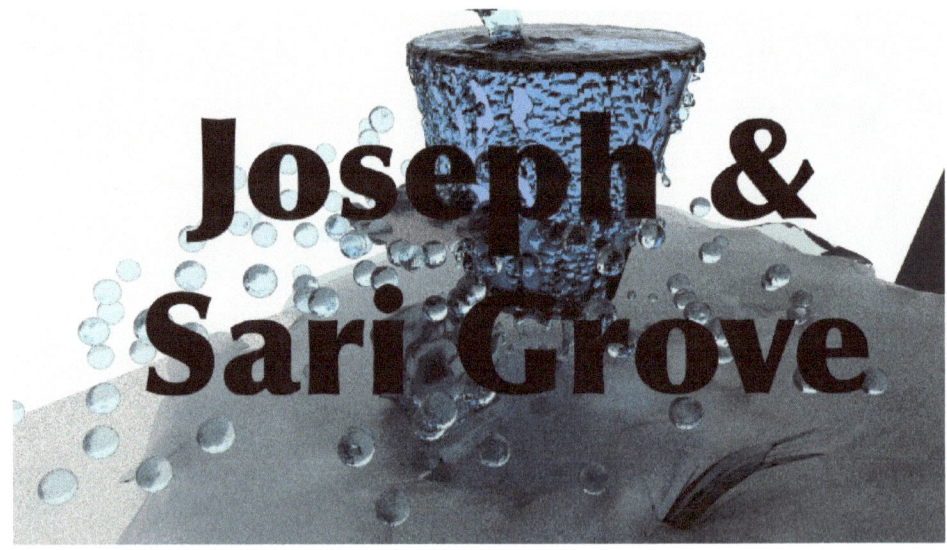

There is a difference between a book of two hundred pages from the very beginning, and a book of two hundred pages which is the result of an original eight hundred pages. The six hundred are there. Only you don't see them. Elie Wiesel

67.

68.

"We are generally the better persuaded by the reasons we discover ourselves than by those given to us by others."
-- Blaise Pascal

69.

70.

He ne'er is crowned with immortality Who fears to follow where airy voices lead. John Keats

71. John 10:7

New International Version (NIV)

7 Therefore Jesus said again, "Very truly I tell you, I am the gate for the sheep.

9 I am the gate; whoever enters through me will be saved.[a] They will come in and go out, and find pasture. 10 The thief comes only to steal and kill and destroy; I have come that they may have life, and have it to the full.

"Not everything you see is a spotted zebra!!!" Joseph would say to me...

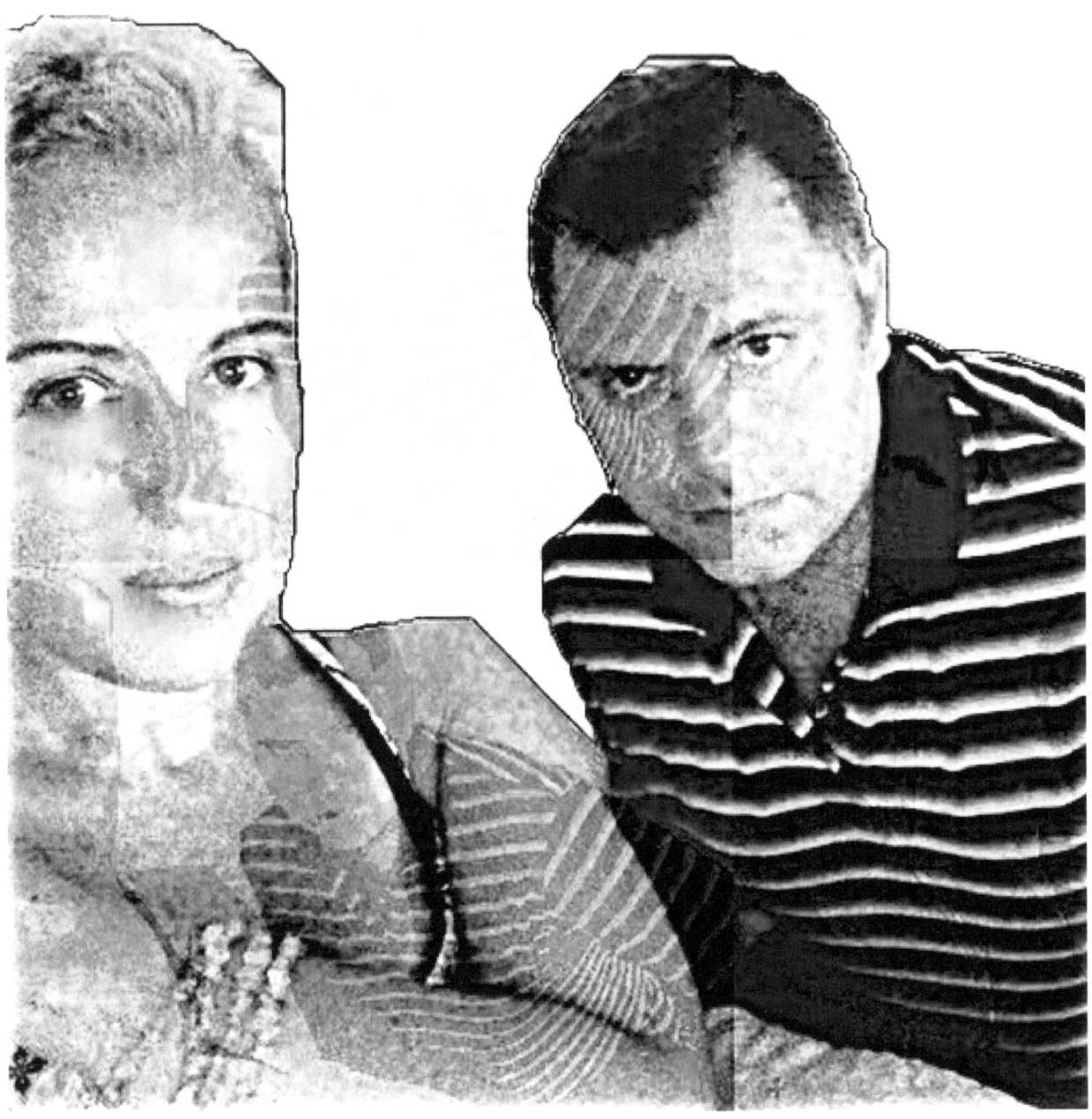

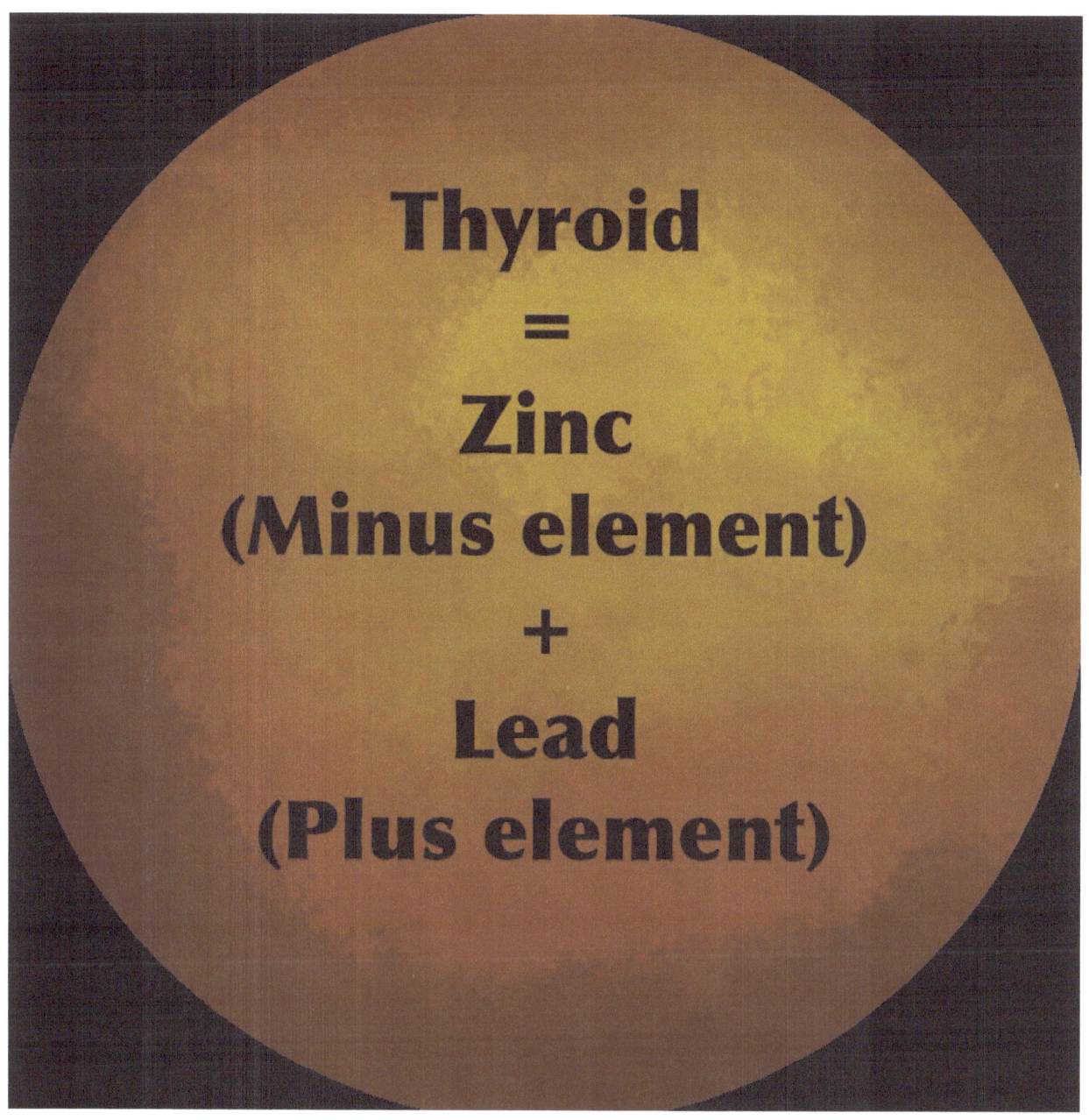

Thyroid=Zinc(Minus element)+Lead(Plus element)

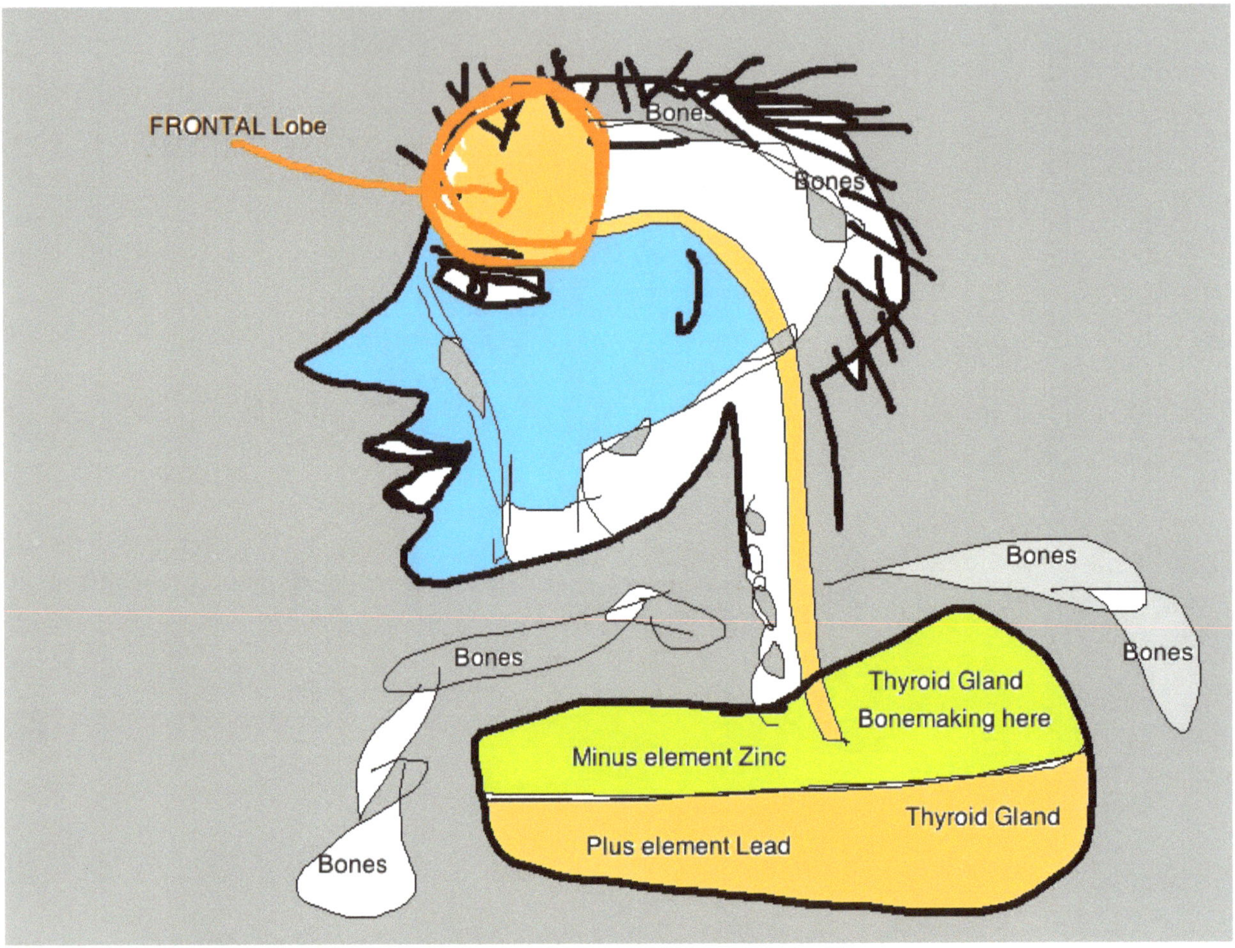

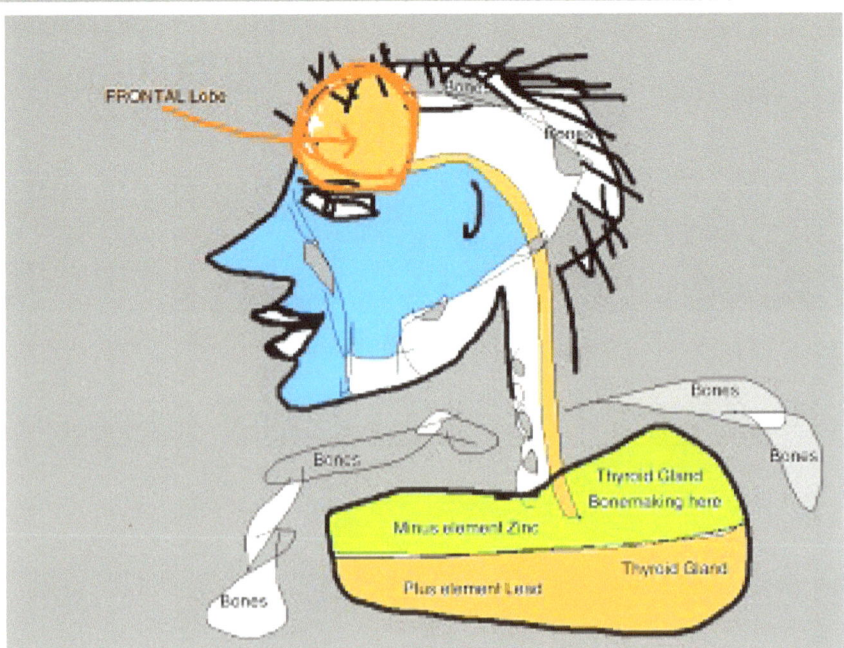

http://www.grovecanada.com/blog/2013/10/frontal-lobe-bones-the-thyroid-gland.html

Thyroid:

Too much Zinc(a Minus Element)=Bipolar, Agent Orange Syndrome, Leprosy, Thalidomide Congenital, Sunburn, Manic, Hysterical, Numbness in Bone, Lack of feeling in fingertips, Muscular Dystrophy, Arthrogryposis(related to Muscular Dystrophy), Peripheral neuropathy-which I say is actually bone damage, hence numbness in fingers or toes as a first indication...(I see nerves as being built in the Kidneys, not the Thyroid by the way-)...
http://en.wikipedia.org/wiki/Phineas_Gage Phineas Gage got a rod stuck through his LEFT FRONTAL Lobe & later exhibited BIPOLAR Zinc Excess symptoms, which shows how the LEFT frontal lobe contains the LEAD element, & the right frontal lobe contains the Zinc element, because if the left frontal lobe is "lost" (or removed), & then Gage started behaving like a bipolar, which is known to be ZINC excess, then that means all he had left was the Zinc side of his frontal lobe, which means the RIGHT side of his frontal lobe...!(Note: Removing a lobe or organ causes a MINUS element excess...DAMAGE to the same organ causes a PLUS element excess...A damaged organ will have like a buildup of gunk, the Plus element...If you just take out a whole Organ, you are left with all the symptoms of a MINUS excess...KNOW this difference!!! ie:remove the Gallbladder causes Magnesium(Minus) excess-so you poop alot, maybe have pain in the joints/cartilage...
A damaged Spleen will have Phosphorus buildup(a Plus element)...Phosphorus is like mold...You may get Parkinson's disease 40 years from the damage occurrence time...Moldy brain...(copper is its opposite & Minus in the Spleen btw)...

Thyroid:

Too much Lead(a Plus Element): Multiple Sclerosis, Sluggishness, Slow Moving...Lupus...Lice...
*read my post about MS & Lupus too...here http://www.grovecanada.com/blog/2013/10/why-are-there-so-many-people-in-saskatchewan-with-multiple-sclerosis.html
*if the right side of the frontal lobe is damaged then behavioral symptoms of Multiple Sclerosis occur which is lead excess because the right side is the Zinc side so damage there reduces zinc thus increasing Lead...
http://www.darenberg.com.au/wine/13/2009-The-Dead-Arm-Shiraz, The Dead arm refers to a fungus that kills off one side of the grape vine in Australia...The other arm lives & the grapes are especially fruity & pungent...One might assume that the Lead element side got fungus, lead is often described as fungus, whilst the other arm of the grapevine is the Zinc arm, which resists fungus well...The dead arm is like Multiple Sclerosis...Too much Lead & it dies...But the other vine, the Zinc side flourishes...Lesson is, in every cloud there is a silver lining!
Scleroderma:I have revised my ideas about Scleroderma, due to its close proximity to Lupus & Multiple Sclerosis, so am now putting Scleroderma into the Lead excess category...
http://www.abstracts2view.com/eular/view.php?nu=EULAR11L_FRI0412 In particular because Scleroderma studies have shown a Vitamin D deficiency, which in my chart is a Zinc element...Since Zinc is opposite to lead in the Thyroid, this confirms(until I am wrong again :( ) that Scleroderma is a LEAD excess ailment...http://www.sclero.org/medical/causes/vitamin-d-deficiency/a-to-z.html This page has links to various studies about Vitamin D deficiency(Zinc deficiency) & scleroderma...(***Comment:Since cigarettes are a Zinc providing drug, one wonders with the current rash of pressure forcing people to quit smoking cigarettes, that, the

few people who actually need that Zinc, people with Multiple sclerosis, Lupus & scleroderma, might have become WORSE By quitting smoking cigarettes...People in dark cold climates also benefit from smoking cigarettes...So, not everyone should be restrained from smoking cigarettes, ESPECIALLY those with Lupus, MS & scleroderma...)
More about scleroderma:
http://www.umich.edu/~snre492/cases_03-04/TarCreek/TarCreek_case_study.htm Tar Creek in Oklahoma, is a mining operation that left that land with severe LEAD EXCESS...The Choctaw Indians from Oklahoma suffer 20 times more scleroderma than a normal population, which points directly at LEAD poisoning as the cause of Scleroderma...(so scleroderma is LEAD excess, like Lupus & Multiple Sclerosis))...
Phototherapy is now the therapy of choice for scleroderma...Since phototherapy is a Zinc based therapy(sunshine & light are Zinc elements), this also confirms that scleroderma is a Lead based excess disorder, since Lead is Zinc's opposite in the Thyroid gland...(on our chart)...

Elements, where to find them in the real world...

Frontal Lobe involvement...Bones...Thyroid...

***Left side Frontal lobe contains Lead, Right side Frontal lobe contains Zinc(THYROID gland)

Thyroid: Zinc (a Minus Element): cigarettes, sunshine, ginger, zinc supplements, Hemimorphite beads...Zinc is called Citrulline malate in bodybuilding supplements, also Niacin or Nicotinamide- these are all in the same family...Vitamin D3 drops fall into the Zinc category too (take these to get rid of toenail fungus which is actually lead poisoning)...Zinc is also found in anti-parasitic drugs like Combantrin (which taken orally get rid of persistent problems like roundworms or pinworms but also seem to rid one of resistant lice problems)...Pyrethrins contain zinc, like
what is found in flea sprays...Wormwood the absinthe herb, is a zinc element too...
Hops the thing they put into beer is also a Zinc element..."Hops" is wormwood is daisies is the active ingredient in Absinthe that kills lice & is "anti-fungal", it is also in the "head" of beer since daisies like to float...Too much Wormwood is also a pesticide, can cause neuro-leptic damage & pain at the back of the neck where the bones start to degrade & compress...Nicotinamide, Niacin is Zinc too...All of these things are different titrations, which means strengths(or weaknesses)...Vincent Van Gogh drank Absinthe, hence the overdose witness...
Combantrin is a Zinc element: see below...

I am 5'10" & very muscular...female...I weigh maybe 191-196 lbs... That said, I needed more than one box of Combantrin...I needed more than two boxes...I am not complaining...The product is brilliant...But if you exercise & eat & take the pills, they may go through you without getting rid of the whole problem...That's just my system, not a fault of the product...So it says don't do more than two rounds...But I needed to do more than two...Also, what I think is that what people are calling lice & bedbugs & roundworms & ringworms, well, they all seem to respond to the same thing...if something is biting your neck like lice, the Combantrin works...If something is stuck on the back of your head like ringworm, Combantrin works...If you have

roundworm in your feces or up your crotch, Combantrin works...You can crush half a pill, put it in some cat food & give it to your cat...It is the same stuff as the veterinary drugs...if your cat is showing lice or bedbugs or fleas or whatever the name is...The sprays seem to be more neuroleptically dangerous than Combantrin...For people & for cats...if you take even one pill less than your body weight needs, you will miss it...Take it later...You can even just chew one if you are feeling buggy but already have enough in your system...Combined with the Well.ca Pedifix funga soap(let it stay on your head or wherever for 10 minutes before rinsing out), you may get bug or worm free...Putting all your soft items into plastic bags helps...Vaccuuming your bed & furniture helps...Roundworm, lice, whatever eggs, are more resistant than before...You really have to go crazy clean to get rid of them...Throw out any item that is suspect that cannot be cleaned...Drop your sugar & iron levels...I also took Wormwood tea, BlackWalnut hull pills, & Clove powder pills...Ginseng tea helps too...D3 drops lift your mood...I even started smoking cigarettes...This type of problem needs a nuclear attack...Combantrin was the best weapon in the arsenal...Thank GOD for Combantrin...Thank God...(Combantrin is called Pyrantel Pamoate as a drug...It turns out I created the lice situation by supplementing with Iron...I know this sounds like an ad for a drug, but if you have ever had to fight lice & found some relief, you will be ecstatically grateful like I was, & am...!)
*Wild rosemary an herbal is also a Zinc element...
Permethrins are all Zinc based elements...
Note:A new homepathic pill, containing wild rosemary as the first ingredient is also a Zinc primary-it is called Mozi-Q, mozi-q.com, & is a pill that makes lice, mosquitos, ticks & other bugs HATE you...(*Mozi-Q, *It also contains other minus elements, including, Zinc, Titanium, Manganese, Iodine & Magnesium-all these MINUS elements in one pill make this pill GREAT!)

More ZINC elements: Turmeric is in the GINGER family...ALL Gingers are in the ZINC family...Zinc is in the sunshine family...Zinc is in the LASER THERAPY family...Zinc is in the PHOTOTHERAPY family...CANADIANS LOVE ZINC THINGS...Buy stock in Turmeric if you are a Canadian...We are cold & live in the dark so we are HIGH in LEAD & LOW in ZINC...You can eat Turmeric powder to get your ZINC...

Meditech is a Laser therapy place in Toronto where you can get laser therapy if you say smashed your kneecap all up & it is swollen & full of fluid & really really hurts...(Cause you fell on the ice because we had a giant power outage at Christmas, & you were getting firewood from the cold freezing cold garage)...True story...Anyways, laser therapy is like getting a whole lot of sunshine on your kneecap...Sunshine is a ZINC...

Phototherapy is the number one choice of treatment for Scleroderma which is another Lead excess problem like Lupus & MS Multiple Sclerosis...

People in Canada like anything in the Zinc family...That is ok, they are right...Even a suntanning booth gives you Zinc...

Vega One the Vegan powder & protein bar company makes a sugar free powder called Energizer(it comes in like straws/small thin packages for $1.69 or so) which I bought at Whole Foods market & wow it has a whole lot of Zinc in it...How do I know? because too much Zinc makes you a little Bipolar...Awake too early in the morning, talk too much, too fast, shopaholic, work like 50 jobs before noon, no hunger, that;s too much Zinc...(Just slow down with Lead things like potatoes, or carrot juice or carrots or...even French/Freedom fries will do...)

Thyroid: Lead (a Plus Element): potatoes, *anti-psychotic drugs like Lithium or Olanzapine Zyprexa or Gabapentin, Carrots, Vitamin A, Yams, Lepidolite beads, Dirt, many anti-seizure drugs are lead based though you should know that Lithium(LI) another element on the Periodic Table acts just like Lead (PL) but is just much much stronger...So Lithium also builds bone like Lead but just faster...'lead pipe water leaded poisoning'-lead pipes cause your water to have extra lead in it which causes or can cause Multiple sclerosis or just real slowness & lack of impulsivity...

CORTISONE shots or hydrocortisone cream, anything in that family are all LEAD ELEMENTS...BUILDS BONE!!!!

Frontal Lobe-Thyroid-Bones

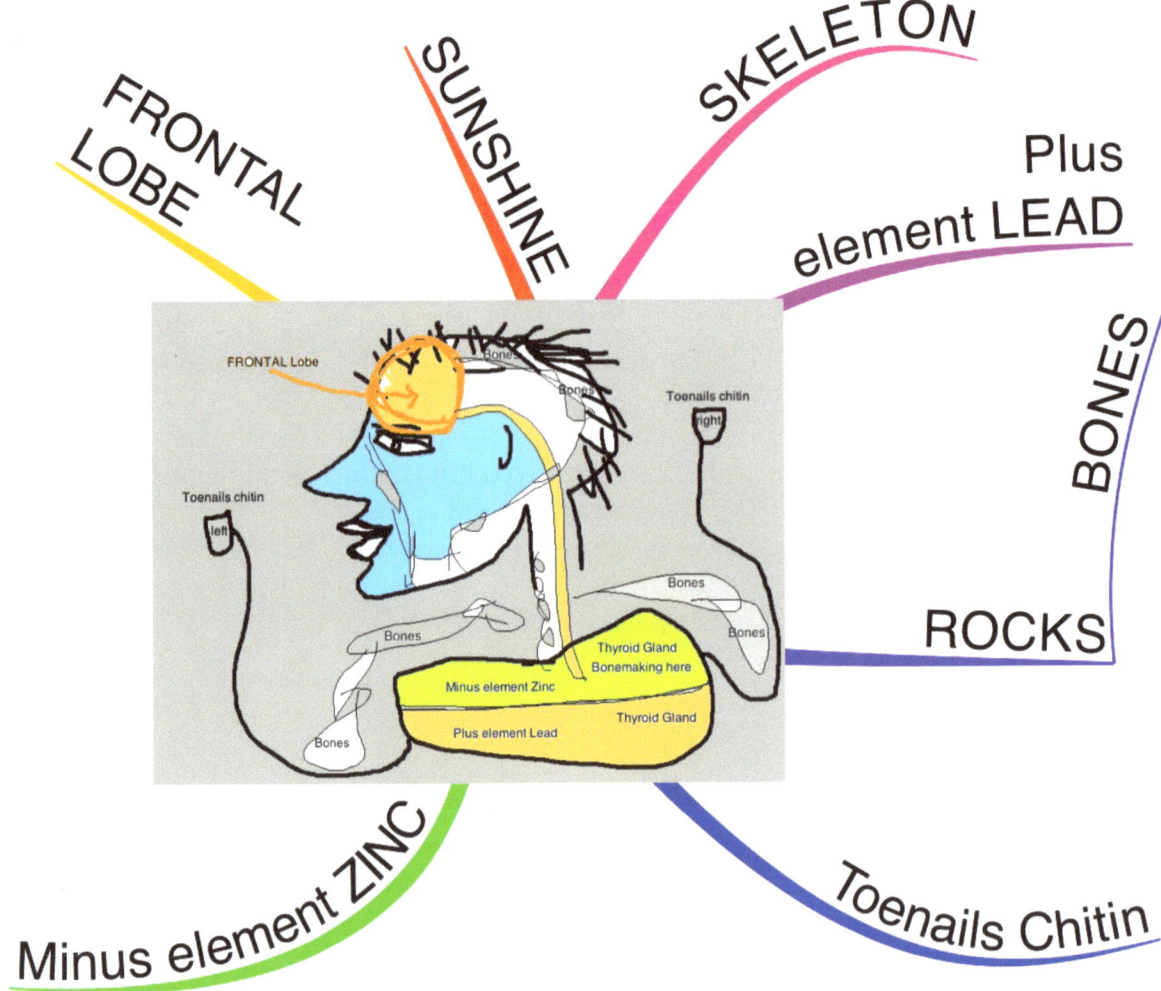

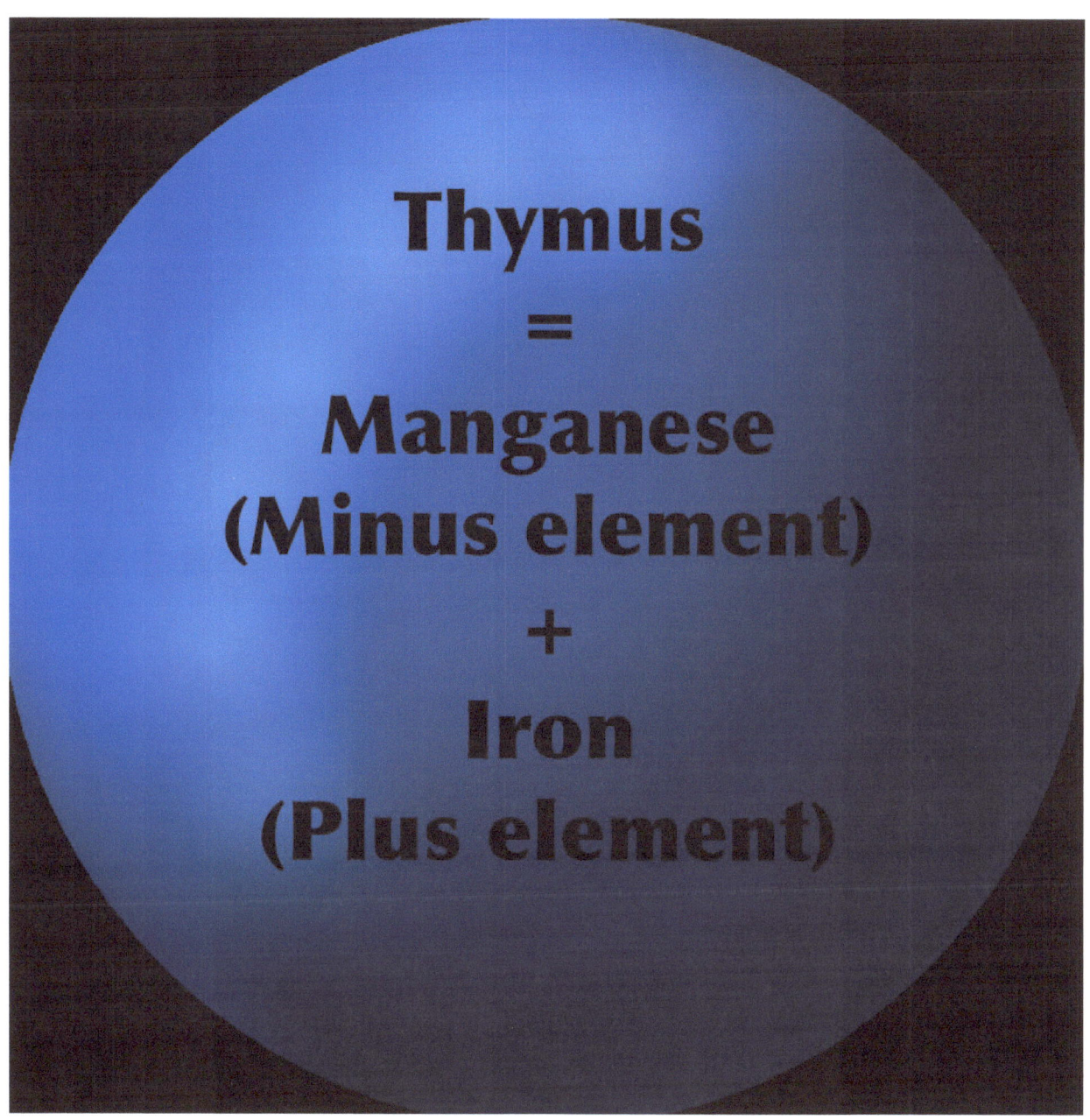

[Thymus=Manganese(Minus element)+Iron(Plus element)](#)

Motor Cortex connects to Thymus which contains Manganese(Minus) & Iron(Plus)

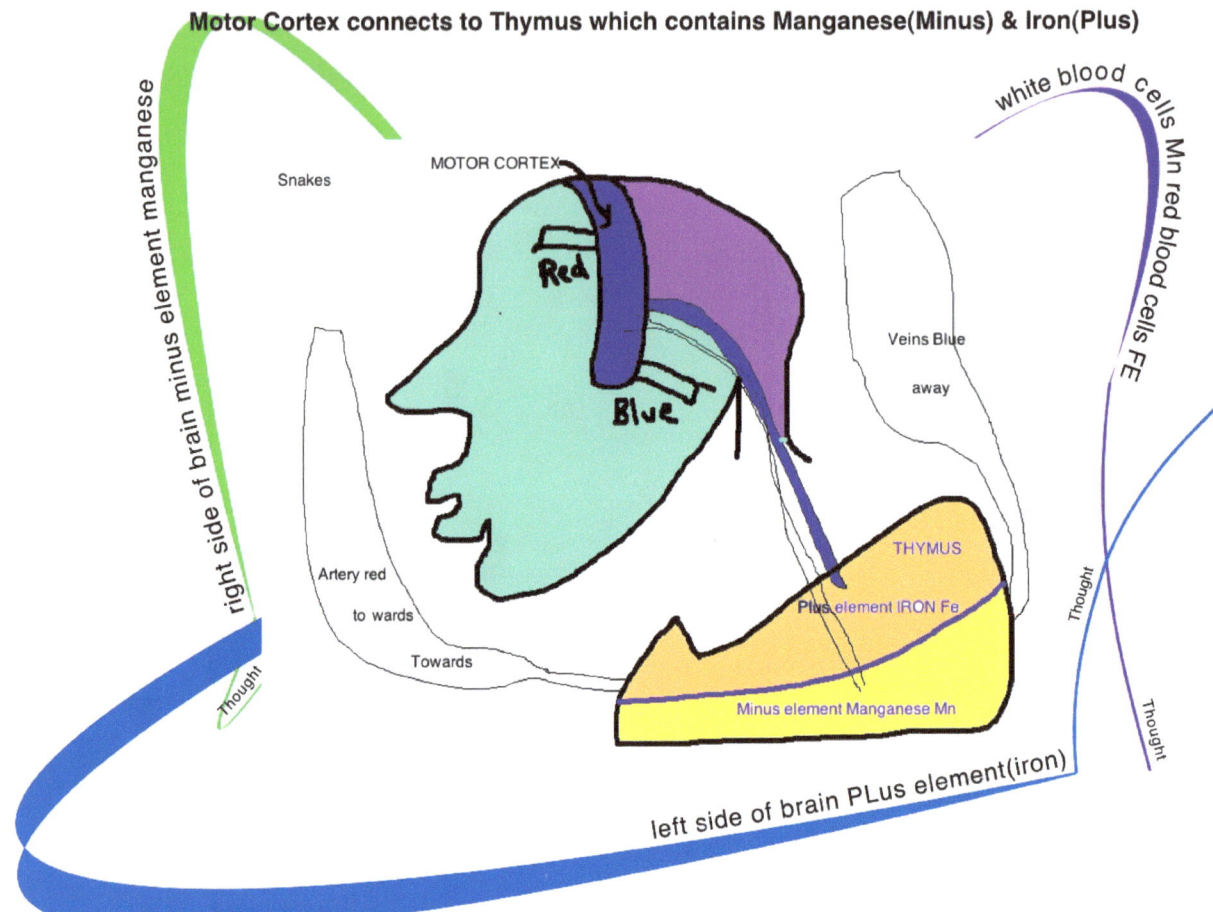

http://www.grovecanada.com/blog/2013/10/motor-cortex-blood-thymus-gland.html

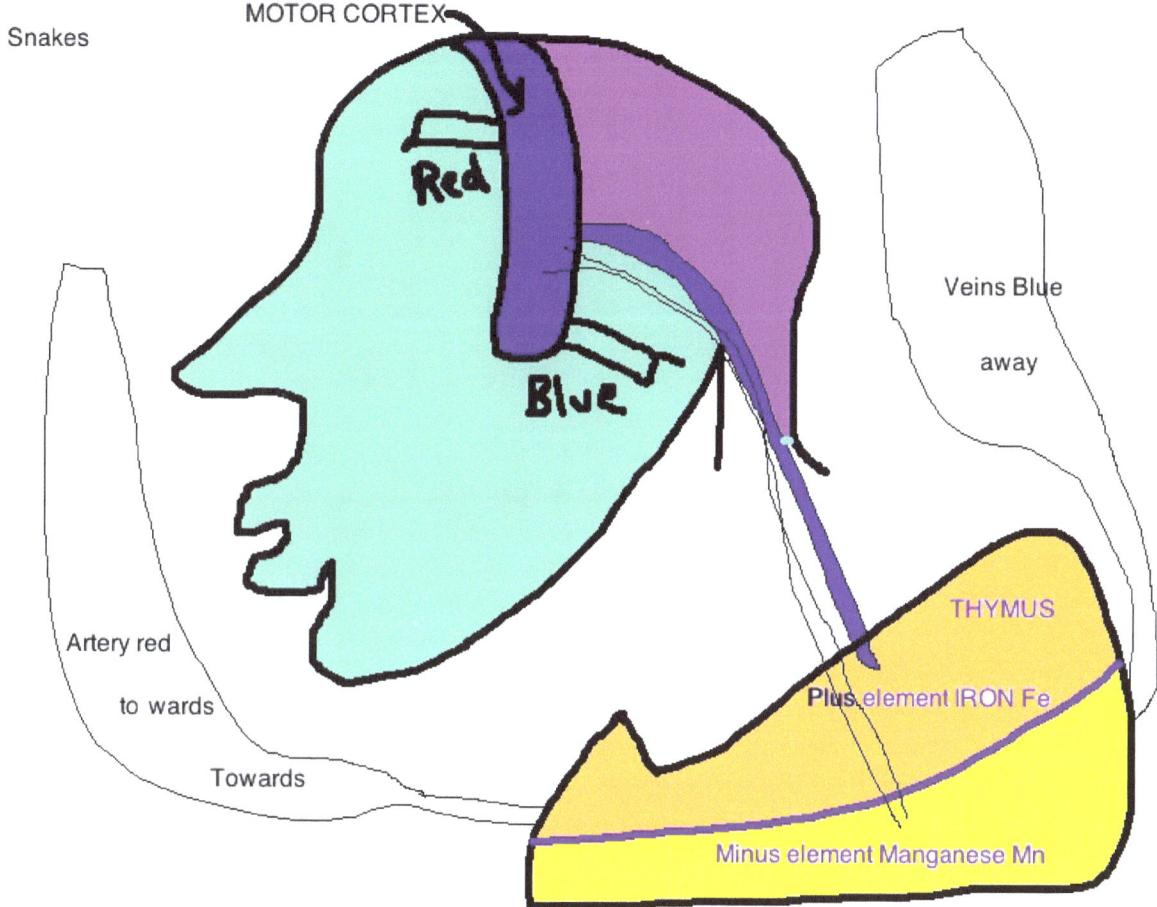

Thymus:

Too much Manganese (a Minus Element): Peanut Allergy, Post Traumatic Stress Disorder with Triggers, Anemia,***PTSD Post traumatic Stress Disorder(playing over the same situation over & over, not moving forward in your life, dwelling on an event from the past),is a Manganese excess(iron deficit)

Signs of PTSD - dwelling on things from the past,going over & over again over the same situation, like your own mental pathways are like a skipping record,*(treat with iron),(hold a pyrite rock in your hand...)
(Go to Ireland-geologically IRON-land...)

Thymus:

 Too much Iron (a Plus Element): Myasthenia Gravis, Hemachromatosis, Particular to Irish people living in "Ire/Iron-land"...

http://www.bioportfolio.com/resources/pmarticle/19873/Severe-Iron-Deficiency-Anemia-And-Lice-Infestation.html

Ok, so the above link points to a study, to find people with severe lice infestation who also had an IRON DEFICIENCY...They only found one(in like a billion)...What that says is that people who get severe lice infestations have TOO MUCH IRON...Which makes sense theoretically too...So if you are suffering from lice, then you should LOWER YOUR IRON levels...(how do you do that? well...you need to add the opposite element to iron in the THYMUS gland...Which is Manganese...***Where to find manganese? I get Black Walnut Hull Powder from Herbies Herbs shop online store, they send it to me, I put a whole bunch 4 tablespoons into whatever I am drinking & stir that with my Hot Straw(hot straws are straws you can use in hot drinks), & sip through the straw...
LICE***Yup, high Iron levels attract lice...So the biggest thing you can do is to add its opposite, manganese into your life...Black Walnut Hull powder is manganese...Put it in your tea-like alot, stir & sip through a straw...Lowers iron making lice not so interested...(you will feel droopy, hungry & maybe faint...But lice will go away)...Also buy a hair clipper from Amazon-I got a Philips one with adjustable comb & can go wireless for like $30 dollars...I set it to 3/8 of an inch & buzzed all my hair off...Then I bleached the whole thing using "Ice Cream" which you buy at Shopper's Drug mart-you choose a tube colour then choose a liquid strength(40% is fine), go home, squirt the tube colour into a plastic dish, mix with equal parts of the liquid hydrogen peroxide, stir with a nylon haired brush, then paint it on your hair...Wait 45 minutes to an hour & presto, your hair is bleached! (neat thing with this method is you can dole out just a bit when roots grow in & total cost is like under 20 dollars for 3 months of home hair bleaching!) Take Mozi-Q or Combantrin tablets while removing lice...Stop all sugars/sulphur, & cut back on Leads(potatoes), cut back on Aluminums(eggs), cut back on Nitrogens(Beets)...Anything on the PLUS element side of my chart, cut back...Anything on the MINUS side , FINE...

More Lice notes & the product called
 "Mozi-Q"...Awesomeness! You can take this as directed, one every hour or so, up to 8, or you can also just take a bunch, & be fine for the rest of the day...I've been taking these after taking Combantrin which is Pyrantel Pamoate...I wanted to switch to something less strong to clear up any final problems...It turns out because I had been taking iron supplements for the past 3 years, that my iron levels were attracting bugs...When I rescued a raccoon & got lice, it was like "Lice, The Movie"...These Mozi-Q pills have been amazing...They taste good, are chewable & really work...If you take them at night, when itchy & scratchy get worse, you actually can sleep...Just a brilliant product...Another thing I did was to lower my iron levels back down...I took Black Walnut Hull powder, which is Manganese, & that lowers your iron levels back down so bugs (lice) don't like you...Mozi-Q actually has 5 different things in it that lower levels in various body parts...The only thing to be careful of is the magnesium(lavender)...Too much magnesium can cause like back pain or soreness & can deplete your heart...It's also a laxative...So you can take Mozi-Q to get rid of lice, for an extended time, but just be aware to slow down or stop if your joints are sore...I also gave two crushed pills to my bengal lady cats, & it totally worked-in their wet food...be aware also that too much, to a cat or a person can cause damage...Less is more when you begin to see how you react...Way better than topical stuff!!(That didn't really work)...Also buying a hair clipper helps(I got a Philips hair clipper & sheared & then bleached my hair)...

Elements:where to find,

Thymus: Manganese (a Minus Element):Peanuts, Peanut butter, Pumpkin Seeds(very strong Manganese actually especially organic pumpkin seeds-eat these if you have lice or bedbug problems to lower your iron levels), Pink Tourmaline beads, Bees, Dr.
Reckeweg R38 R39 tinctures (these tinctures remove ovarian cysts-right & left ovary) (Manganese causes detachment of the cyst)...Manganese is also found in Black walnut hulls which help one to rid the body of parasites(including lice problems)....Manganese is also found in Almond extract...Peanuts are nuts that grow in the ground, whereas Walnuts are tree nuts...ground nuts will have more manganese than tree nuts-hence the fact that people with nut allergies Can be non-allergic to walnuts but allergic to peanuts-it is the Manganese they are allergic to...(Manganese lowers iron...which is why they give you an iron shot when you have a reaction...)
*Cedron an herbal is also a Manganese element...
**Walnut leafs are also a Manganese element...

Thymus: Iron (a Plus Element): Pyrite beads, Iron supplements, B12, Red meats, Pink meats, White meats, Dark meats, Marcasite rocks

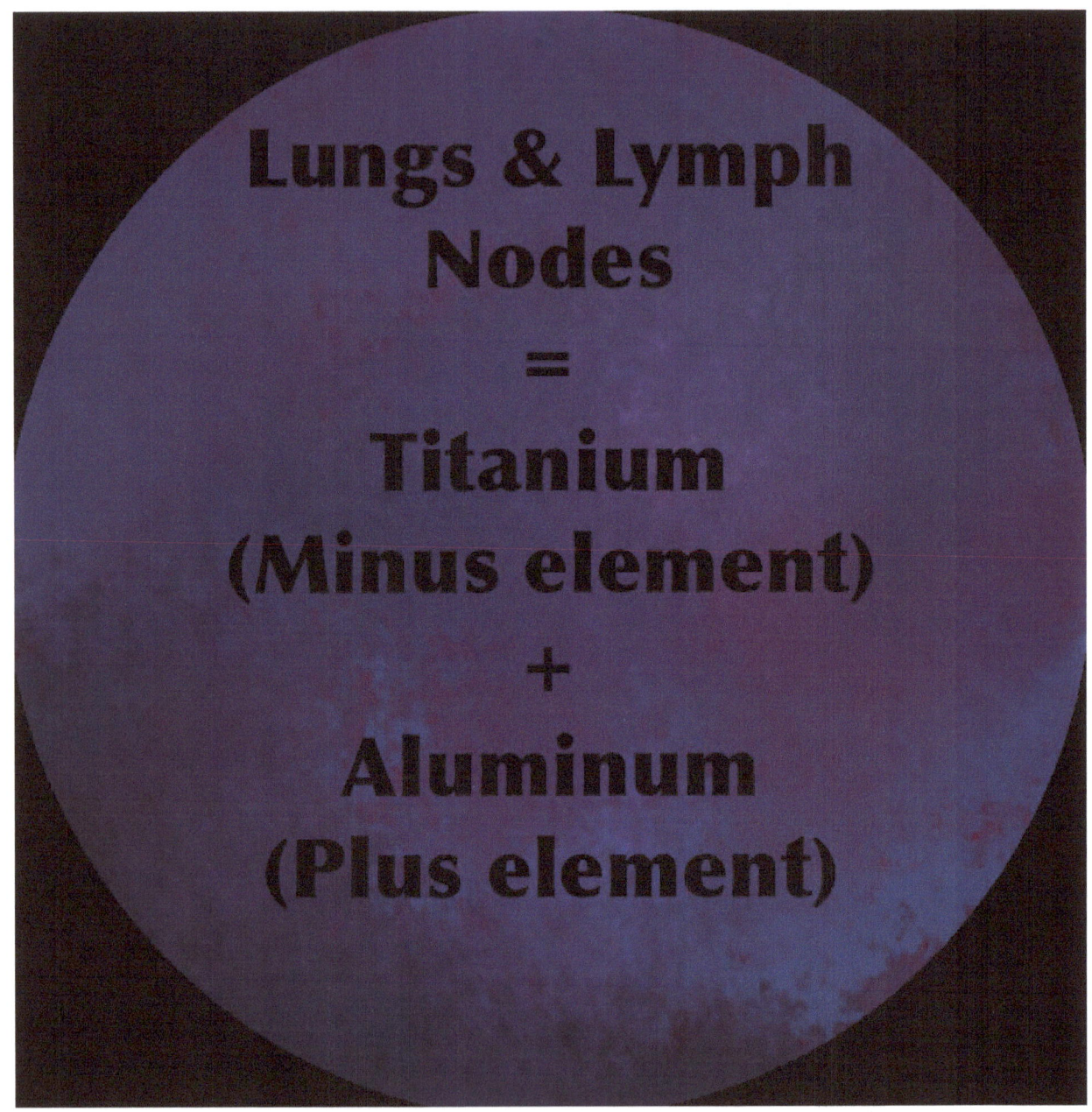

Lung & Lymph Nodes=Titanium(Minus element)
+Aluminum(Plus element)

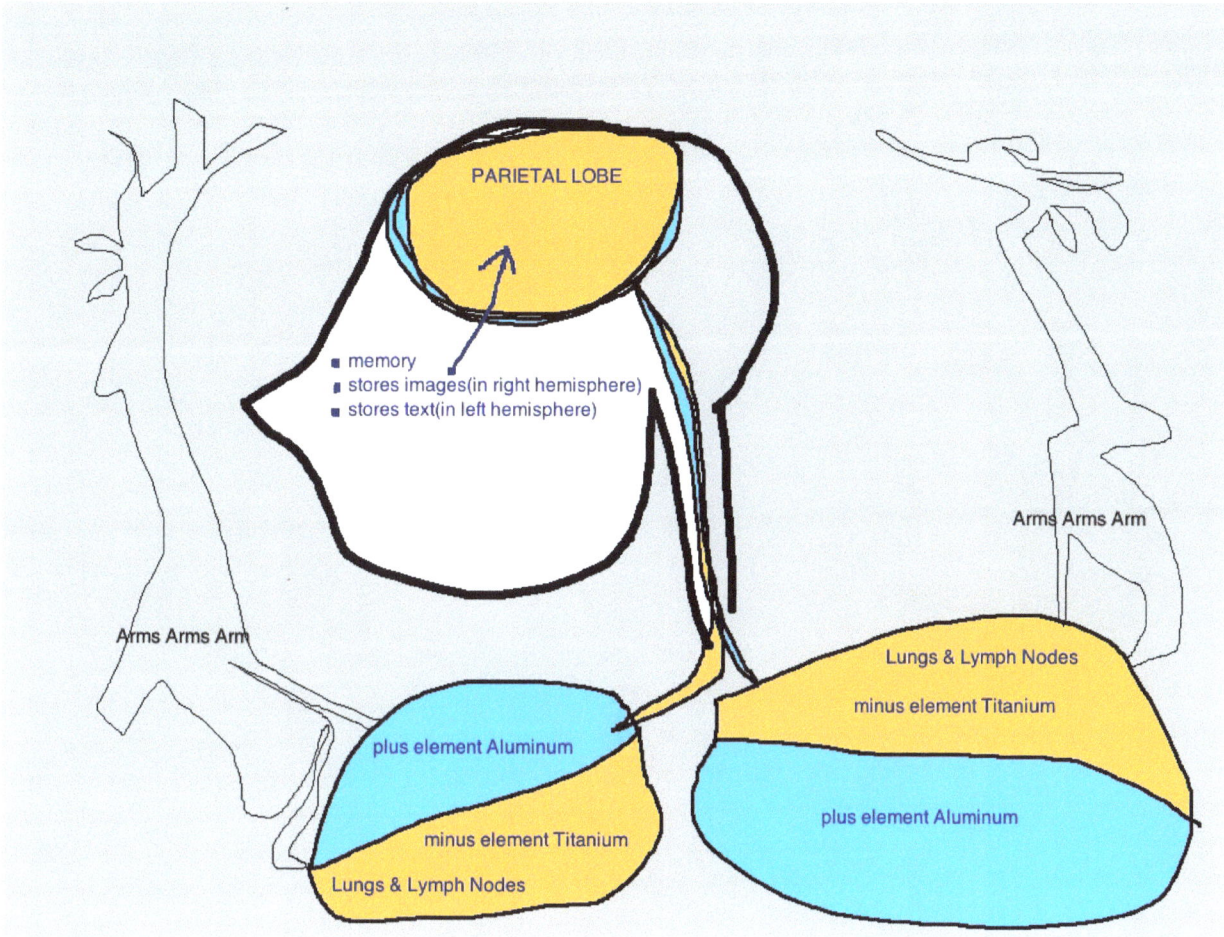

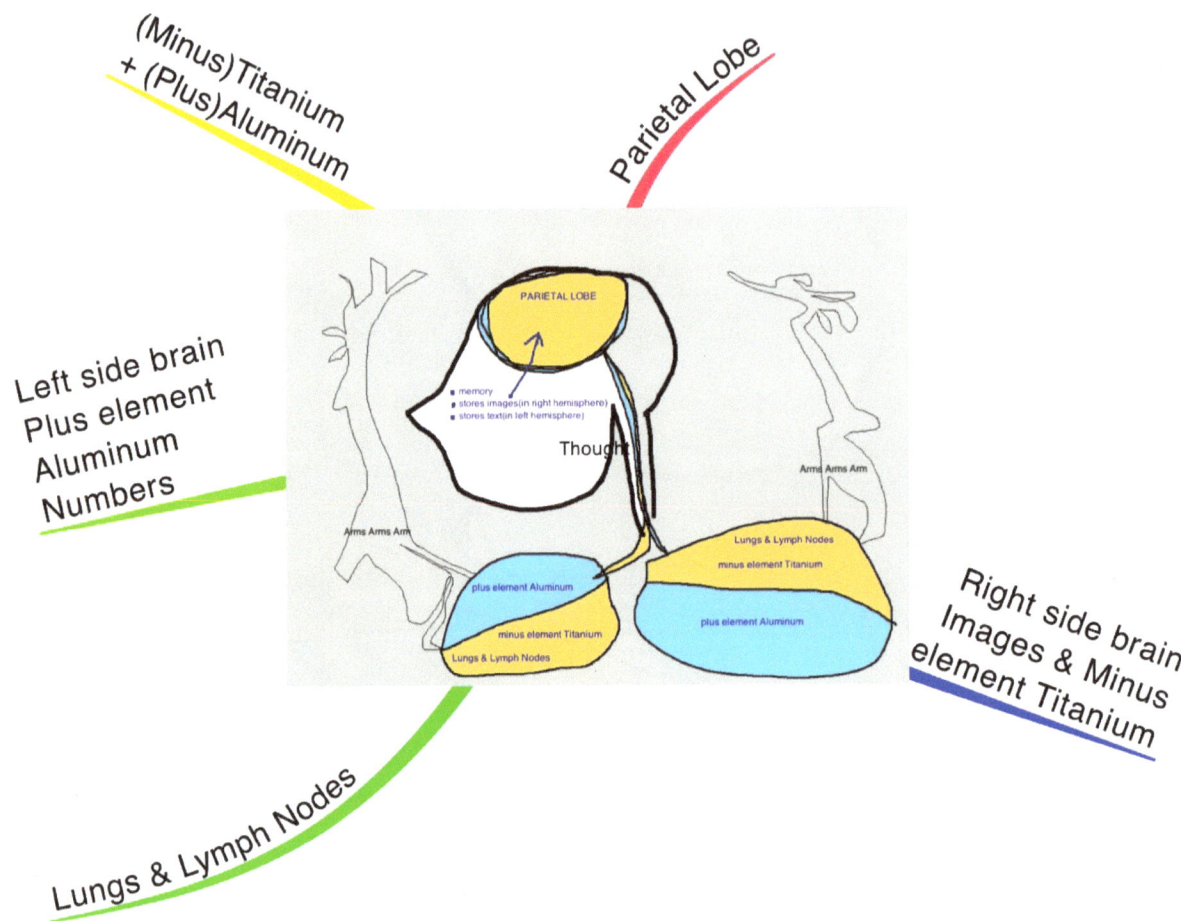

http://www.grovecanada.com/blog/2013/10/parietal-lobe-lungs-lymph-nodes-memory.html

Lungs Lymph Nodes

= Too much Titanium (a Minus Element): Alzheimer's, Schizophrenia, Fear Panic Anxiety (Attacks), Memory Loss short medium or long term, Cerebral Palsy congenital, Hyperhidrosis/Sweatyness, Amnesia
Note:Anxiety is actually related to memory loss, as are panic attacks-yo are trying to do a task or plan your day, say while driving to work, & you are having trouble remembering all the tasks you need to do, then the anxiety begins, later it can develop into a panic attack-it is a fear that you cannot perform-this is all a Titanium excess in the Lung Lymph Node system...
PLEASE VISIT GROVECANADA.COM & TYPE ALZHEIMER'S IN TO THE SEARCH BOX TO FIND ALL MY POSTS ON THIS SUBJECT THERE(or see the links below)...ESPECIALLY TO

EXPLAIN WHY TITANIUMS ARE A MEMORY STEALER, & ALUMINUMS ARE MEMORY BOOSTERS...

(Doctors usually say the opposite because they have NOT accounted for the fact that people with asthma & other Aluminum EXCESS problems SELF-MEDICATE with Titanium asthma drugs, thus CAUSING their own memory loss...Later when pathologists examine the brain, they find aluminum deposits because that is from the initial CAUSE of the reason they OVERMEDICATED with asthma Titanium memory loss drugs...

Concussion, Traumatic brain Injury, Alzheimer's: - The Grove Body ...

Jan 31, 2013 ... Two things I want to say right off about traumatic brain injury: 1)Potassium levels RISE when injury happens...Rise...Too much potassium can ...

http://www.grovecanada.com/blog/2013/01/concussion-traumatic-brain-injury-alzheimers.html

The Grove Body Part Chart...: Weblogs

Sep 6, 2013 ... The reason people find that the brains of people with Alzheimer's contain Aluminum is that yes indeed there was Aluminum there...BUT THAT ...

http://www.grovecanada.com/blog/weblogs/

The Grove Body Part Chart...: Aluminum, Titanium, & Lungs ...

Oct 14, 2013 ... All these Titanium things can cause memory loss & Alzheimer's disease as well as schizophrenia...On a low level, Titanium things thin the ...

http://www.grovecanada.com/blog/aluminum-titanium-lungs-lymphatic-system-nodes/

Lungs & Lymph Nodes:

Too much Aluminum (a Plus Element): Tuberculosis, Cystic Fibrosis, Asthma...Warnings:People with Asthma(an Aluminum excess) often overmedicate their asthma medications(which are Titanium based), causing severe memory loss & even Alzheimer's disease...be forewarned! Asthma meds cause memory loss, as do all statins, aspirins & marijuana drugs...Everything in balance...

***Pulmonary Hypertension resembles Tuberculosis...It is also excess Aluminum though the aspect of infection on top of the Aluminum needs to be cleared up as well(Infection is in the Pancreas & is a Sulphur excess that you treat with Selenium elements like antibiotics or garlic-raw garlic is stronger)...

*Eczema correlates strongly with people who have asthma & as well with people who have egg allergies-we know asthma is an aluminum excess, we know eggs are an aluminum element, so we can now point out that Eczema is also an Aluminum excess...A further confirmation is that Chamomile cream, a Titanium element, works very well as a treatment for eczema...Titanium, being the opposite to Aluminum, confirms our ideas...

(**if you are trying to figure out what something is, that is a pattern-how I figured out eczema above...See if the imbalance correlates to other things that you already know the answer to, then form a hypothesis, then check to see if treatments are correct according to your hypothesis...Another clue will be contraindications-something that contraindicates with a drug will be similar or the same-if you are trying to understand or figure out a herbal form of whatever drug you are investigating...)

A recent article on WDDTY (What Doctor's Don't Tell You), explains that most people don't need to be taking statin drugs for their heart...Those at risk(for heart events) are those not with high cholesterol levels but those with RAISED CALCIUM levels in their ARTERIES...Apparently current protocols for prescribing these statin drugs(like Crestor or Lipitor or even aspirins) are being revised to reflect this new information... http://www.wddty.com (though, let's be honest, raised calcium levels needs Iodine if you are going to get specific...Get a Vinpocetine(iodine) supplement & get rid of that calcium in your arteries more directly than the Titanium the statin gives...

Elements where to find them...

Lungs Lymph Nodes: Titanium (a Minus Element): Cannabis, Aspirin, Birch Bark, Statin drugs, Crestor, Lipitor, Rutile crystal beads, Comfrey, Mint, Chamomile tea, (*weird thing:Paper can be laced with Titanium, like hash oil using Benzene Carbon to stick, making people "suggestible" to the text)...! Titanium is also found in Clove supplements, which are the third part of a three part anti-parasitic treatment...(the 3 part anti-parasite treatment is Wormwood, Black Walnut Hulls & Cloves-which are all Minus elements- Zinc, Manganese, Titanium...Minus elements remove things from the body that
are unwanted...
Lowering your lead, iron & aluminum levels is a way to get rid of parasites/lice...Which is why people with sickle cell anemia don't get malaria-bugs don't like people with low iron levels...Unfortunately, low iron levels can cause mental problems-but at least you are

Grove Brain Part Chart

Brain Parts 12	Minus Element -F	Plus Element +M
Link to Body Part Chart	chromosomes female	chromosomes male
Holistic	Detoxify	Nutrify
Frontal lobe	Zinc -1	Lead =12
Motor Cortex	Manganese -2	Iron +11
Parietal Lobe	Titanium -3	Aluminum +10
Medulla Oblongata	Potassium -4	Gold +9
Pons	Carbon +5	Nitrogen +8
Occipital Lobe	Selenium -6	Sulphur +7
Cerebellum	Oxygen -7	Hydrogen +6
Pituitary Gland	Iodine -8	Calcium +5
Globus Palladus & Hypothalamus	Copper -9	Phosphorus +4
Broca's Area & Wernicke's area	Magnesium -10	Mercury +3
Temporal Lobe	Fluorine -11	Bismuth +2
Corpus Callosum & Cerebral Aqueduct	Boron -12	Molybdenum +1

bug free! (PTSD is low iron btw)... **(Note: Grove Brain Part Chart is new for 2015-it contains 24 chromosomes, of which, for example, Bismuth would be chromosome 22...**

Heroin is a painkiller in the Fluorine group...Too much of any painkiller can stop your heart...Think of sleeping pills, a Titanium group(can put you to sleep for good)...

Comment about epilepsy:many people think that marijuana a Titanium is good for epilepsy...Now if you look at heroin, a Fluorine, you may know that in the case of an overdose, injecting saltwater can reverse the danger & save the person's life...Now many people know that RAISING salt levels in an epileptic can help them remain seizure free for life...So think about it...If heroin LOWERS salt levels, then that is bad for an epileptic...Marijuana, a less strong Minus element Titanium than heroin a very very strong Fluorine(on the Grove Body & Grove Brain Parts Charts the Minus elements get stronger as you descend down the body so Titaniums are much weaker detoxifiers than Fluorines like Heroin), will also LOWER salt levels...meaning in the long term it is going to cause problems for an epileptic...So my position is that marijuana is bad for epilepsy...On the other hand, the way that Titanium drugs help you to forget things(they cause memory loss) can be soothing to someone who is troubled...That forgetting can be helpful to someone who is sad about their life...So psychologically, Titanium drugs may make someone "feel" better, even if it is making

their condition worse...Like eating chocolate cake may make the obese person feel happier, though it is not helping their causal condition...But not to be discredited!
Anti-histamines are Titaniums
*Titaniums make you sweatier & more forgetful...
PINE BARK is a Titanium...So is mint...

***For pulmonary hypertension, tuberculosis, Or any major lung breathing problem you need to treat withTitaniums for the root cause, but also Seleniums to get rid of the infection...Imagine a piece of cement lodged in your lung that later becomes infected...You take seleniums, like antibiotics or raw garlic, to remove the infection, THEN you need to dissolve the lump of cement which is Aluminum, which can be done with Titanium things...At this strength of problem you need a strong Titanium like- ORGANIC VIRGIN UNREFINED HEMP SEED OIL (which can be put on salad-keep it cold don't heat this oil)...Opium is a strong Titanium...Morphine is a strong Titanium...(Note:Titaniums can cause memory loss...Also, sometimes the Titanium is not strong enough to dissolve the cement aluminum dust-at that point you may need a surgeon to go in & try to remove any lumps or clumps, which can be dangerous...try some very strong titaniums first in rotation, see which one you like, then take breaks to evaluate if it worked & if you are losing your memory...Once the infection is gone, cleared up by antibiotics or religiously eating raw garlic(really)(it is easier to eat raw garlic cloves in plain Greek yogurt by the way-Christo used to eat this for lunch, made by Jeanne-Claude his wife)...Anyways, once the infection is gone you do need the Titaniums whichever one you choose to rid the lung of the inhaled cement dust...Cement dust, being Aluminum, is a prime causative problem for breathing troubles across the board...Pulmonary Hypertension is most likely a renamed form of Tuberculosis, renamed so that people won't freak out...TB is a really scary word...(Lung Cancer by the way is a Cancer/Calcium excess-see the Adrenal Gland to cure that...clue:Iodine things help...Fish & seaweed contain iodine, as does Nettle Leaf tea...)

Lungs & Lymph Nodes: Aluminum (a Plus Element): Bauxite is a rock & a Bead, Cement, Arnica Pills, Cinnamon/echinacea, Chocolate-Arnica Pills are excellent for fixing memory loss (I think they have great promise for Alzheimer's)...Aloe, Agave is in tequila, Witch Hazel, Anti-Perspirants, Calendula/Marigolds...Wax is an aluminum element, as is Bubble Tea (those tapioca bubbles are made from turnips! Excellent memory builders!)*Sage leaf contains piles of memory building Aluminum-not only that but sage leaf has been found in clinical studies to improve memory loss problems in patients with Alzheimer's disease...Sage leaf also reduces sweatyness, because of course, things with Aluminum are styptic & sweat-stifling! Sage would also help heal scar tissue up...or heal wounds...(Sage leaf tincture is about 16$ at Whole Foods market)(Yes it works!)(My sweaty husband is taking it, & now not so sweaty!)(I liked him sweaty btw, it was his decision)...
Sage leaf tea(Get the herb Sage then add boiled water to a French press, let it steep, then squish down the press & pour...), Sage leaf tea works great for cracked heels(I learnt,while at McGill University, that tea & coffee can be mixed together & drunk as one drink-Based on that, I put my Sage herb into my French Press with my coffee grinds-herb tea can be a little dull in the mornings)(Note:A hand crank coffee bean grinder makes for awesome upper body work-outs)...

(Back to the cracked heel)A cracked heel is actually an Aluminum deficiency...So Sage, as an Aluminum, heals up that muscle tissue there, fast, like any good Aluminum/Cholesterol thing might...(creams don't really work for cracked heels, but smell nice)...

Histadine(a precursor to Histamine is an Aluminum element)(both are AL)(AL is aluminum)...

 Aloe Vera Gel: Aloe is in the Aluminum family...Yes, it heals wounds, builds muscle, increases memory...One thing women who have children will like is that Aloe Vera gel(you drink it) will repair the muscle tissue in droopy breasts...It is also a memory enhancer for people with Alzheimer's disease which is a Titanium excess...

Chai tea is an Aluminum...

Again, ARNICA in all its forms, topical or pills, is a memory boosting Aluminum...

Eggs are in the aluminum family too...They often call it "cholesterol" when referring to eggs...Which is why you get a Titanium as a "cholesterol lowerer"...Notice your memory loss on that cholesterol lowering pill? That's the sign of a Titanium drug...

Yes Chocolate falls into the Aluminum category!

***Chocolate update Mon. Dec. 9, 2013 11:44 am: We ate a pile of SUGAR-FREE chocolates gotten from Shopper's Drug Mart in the secret sugar-free section there...The Aluminum factor in chocolate restores memory but also be aware that Aluminum things make one poop alot... (understatement)! The Potassium in the sugar-freeness, the art. sweeteners will make someone like myself a little dizzy, since K Potassium lowers blood pressure...But good for a high blood pressure person to take...

*Sage Leafs or Sage leaf tinctures, sage, is an Aluminum element...(totally stops sweatyness! If you are menopausal or just sweaty...also boosts memory)... SAGE LEAF TEA!

Topical Arnica cream is also a great Aluminum element...

Mayonnaise(eggs) is another Aluminum element...(memory booster)

After much deliberation, I am putting those empty gelatin capsules, the thing that goes AROUND your medicine pills, as well as the stuff that holds your medicine powders together, into the ALUMINUM category of elements...So the NON-medicinal ingredient of whatever pill or capsule you take, which is made of gelatin, is an ALUMINUM thing...(Beef tallow which is what the base of bird suet is, is also an aluminum element-which gave me the clues for gelatin capsules)...

72. http://www.neuroskills.com/brain-injury/parietal-lobes.php (I used this link AFTER I developed my theory about the right & left sides of the Parietal lobe, in order to see, to check, IF my ideas were at all concurrent with other researchers current thinking...But I did not & do not GET my ideas from other people's work...Which is why I only check

AFTER deciding what my own thoughts are first...!This is an important distinction between original research & thought & derivate copying...)

73. The Lungs & Lymph Nodes in the BRAIN...

74. THE PARIETAL LOBE:If the left frontal lobe is the Lead(plomb) element, & the right Frontal lobe is the Zinc element, THEN one might posit the RIGHT PARIETAL lobe (Lung & lymph node system) is the TITANIUM element, & the LEFT PARIETAL lobe is the Aluminum system...Seeing as the PLUS elements line up on the Grove Body Part Chart, & the Minus ones too...(Aluminum & Lead are both PLuses...)

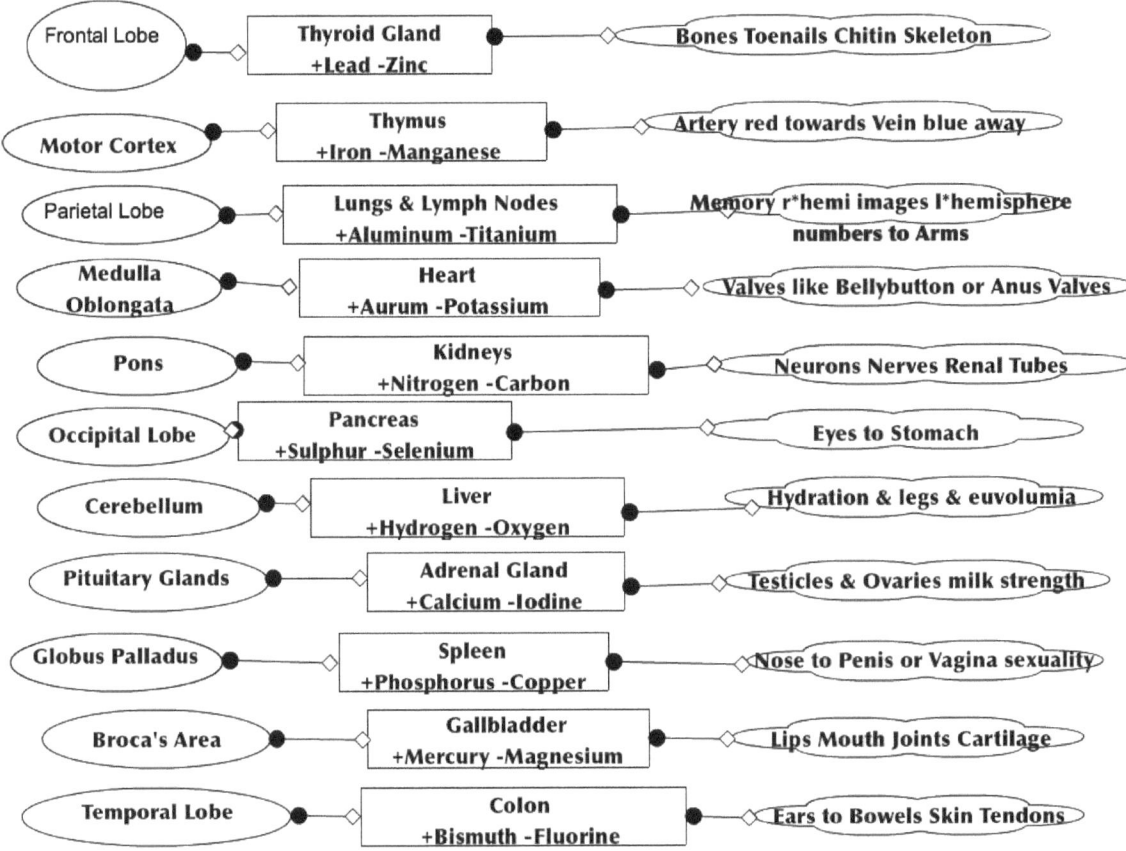

Frontal Lobe	Thyroid Gland +Lead -Zinc	Bones Toenails Chitin Skeleton
Motor Cortex	Thymus +Iron -Manganese	Artery red towards Vein blue away
Parietal Lobe	Lungs & Lymph Nodes +Aluminum -Titanium	Memory r*hemi images l*hemisphere numbers to Arms
Medulla Oblongata	Heart +Aurum -Potassium	Valves like Bellybutton or Anus Valves
Pons	Kidneys +Nitrogen -Carbon	Neurons Nerves Renal Tubes
Occipital Lobe	Pancreas +Sulphur -Selenium	Eyes to Stomach
Cerebellum	Liver +Hydrogen -Oxygen	Hydration & legs & euvolumia
Pituitary Glands	Adrenal Gland +Calcium -Iodine	Testicles & Ovaries milk strength
Globus Palladus	Spleen +Phosphorus -Copper	Nose to Penis or Vagina sexuality
Broca's Area	Gallbladder +Mercury -Magnesium	Lips Mouth Joints Cartilage
Temporal Lobe	Colon +Bismuth -Fluorine	Ears to Bowels Skin Tendons

Note:The first element on the cover chart above is the Plus, all the way down...The second one is the Minus...(If I am right , that explains that the Titanium right Parietal lobe controls the left side of the body, the "artistic side" the IMAGES side, & the Aluminum element LEFT side of the Parietal lobe controls the numbers side, the accountant in all of us...

75. Ok...I am right...The LEFT SIDE OF THE PARIETAL LOBE IS THE ALUMINUM SIDE...
76. THE RIGHT SIDE OF THE PARIETAL LOBE IS THE TITANIUM SIDE...
77. THUS DAMAGE TO THE LEFT SIDE PARIETAL LEADS TO MEMORY LOSS...
78. DAMAGE TO THE RIGHT SIDE PARIETAL LOBE LEADS TO ASTHMA...
79. MORE FAMILIAR IS THAT DAMAGE TO LEFT SIDE PARIETAL MUCKS UP YOUR NUMBERS SYSTEM...(LEFT SIDE CONTROLLING NUMBERS & RIGHT HAND)...

80. DAMAGE TO RIGHT SIDE PARIETAL LEADS TO SPATIAL DRAWING ARTSY LEFT HANDED SKILLS BEING LOST...(RIGHT HEMISPHERE CONTROLLING ARTSY THINGS)...

81. Now that we have confirmation that Aluminum is on left side parietal & titanium is on right side parietal, thus PLUS element on left side of brain, Minus element on right side of brain, we can now continue to formulate theories for the rest of the brain parts...

82.

83. So far, we know both the frontal lobe(thyroid), & parietal lobe(lungs & lymph nodes), both agree with the theory that the LEFT side of the brain contains the PLUS elements, & the RIGHT side contains the MINUS elements...

84. We could maybe guess that holds true all the way along?

85. (**Remember, we know the left side of the brain controls the right side of the body & vice versa, all the way through!)

86.

87. Book 1 is: GROVE BODY PART CHART:A MEDICAL ARTS INNOVATION(EACH ORGAN CONTAINS 2 OPPOSING ELEMENTS)

88. http://addictions.about.com/od/dailylifewithaddiction/a/What-Is-In-Heroin.htm

89.

90. More Titanium elements: These are all in the Titanium category...Heroin, Poppy flower, Poppyseeds, Opium, Morphine...

91. Warning:Heroin, though it comes from the Poppy Flower, is often cut with other things...So your Heroin could be cut with: Methamphetamine(a Copper which causes rushing, accidents & bad decisions), Local Anaesthetics(a Fluorine which is a paralytic & rape drug), Black Shoe Polish(it smells like tar, so they fake the black tar heroin smell with shoe polish-a very dangerous Hydrogen is my best guess), Quinine(which is a Selenium, like garlic or antibiotics or insulin, can cause hypoglycemia or lack of Sulphur or Sugar in the Pancreas), Strychnine which is a rat poison & can make you bleed out, have dementia, or develop symptoms of Grave's disease, anorexia)...

92. So before you buy your Heroin ASK THE DEALER:"What exactly exactly exactly is this CUT with???"...Get an ingredient list...You wouldn't eat at McDonald's without the ingredient list, why buy Heroin without one? p.s. most of the time Heroin is illegal...So be prepared to go to jail...Because you will be going...

93.

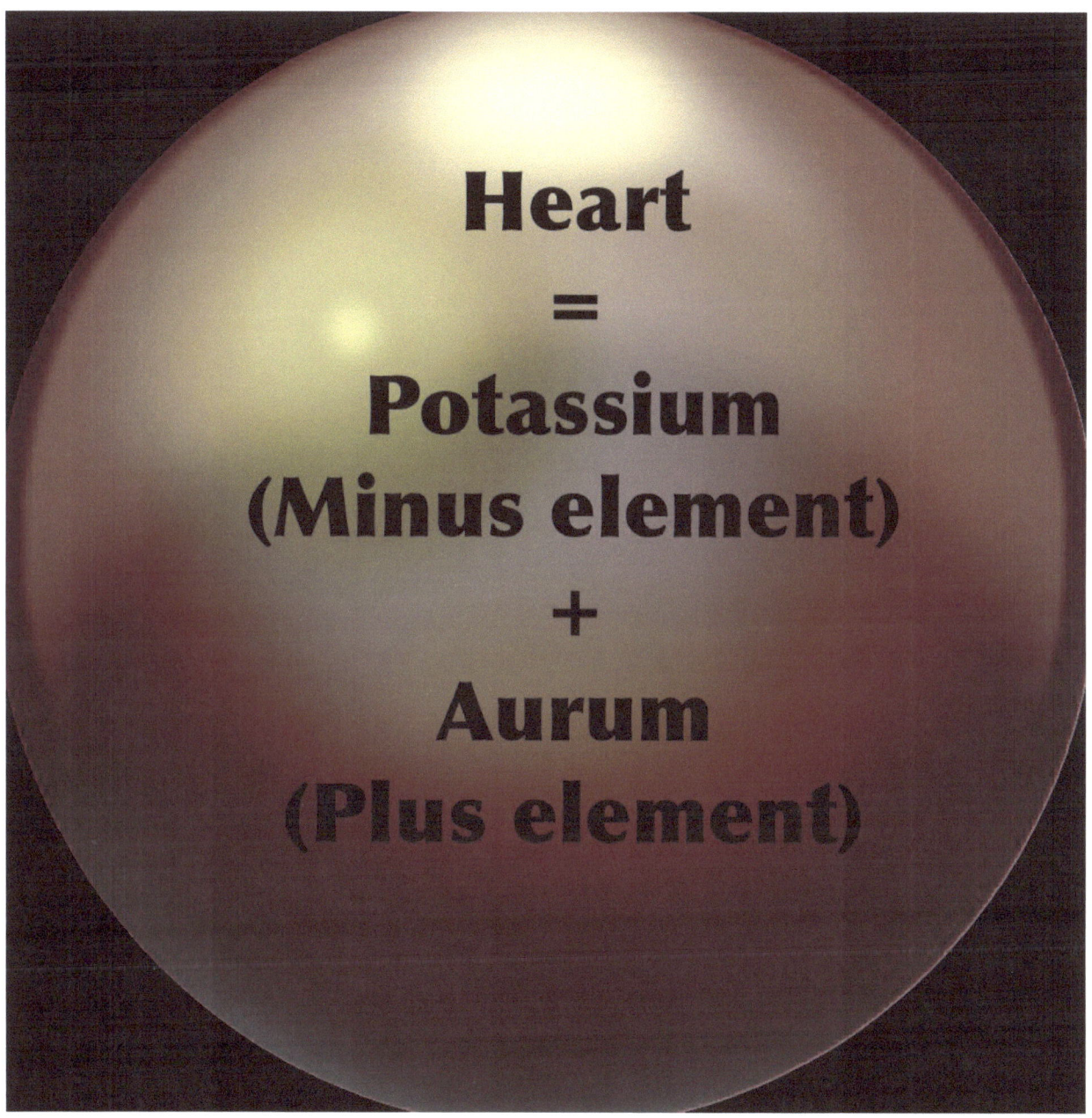

Heart=Potassium(Minus element)+Aurum(Plus element)

http://www.grovecanada.com/blog/2013/10/medulla-oblongata-heart-blood-pressure.html

Heart to Brain stem & Minus element is Potassium, PLus element is Aurum

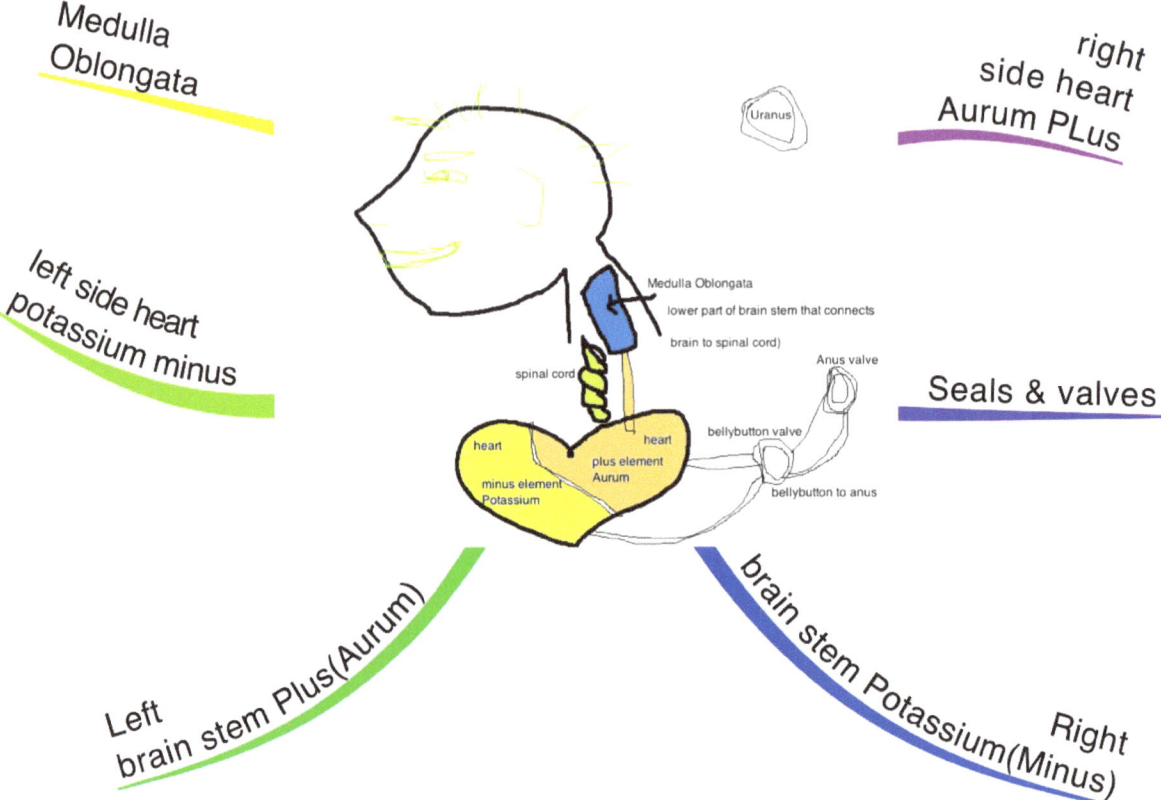

Medulla
Oblongata

right
side heart
Aurum PLus

left side heart
potassium minus

Seals & valves

Left
brain stem Plus(Aurum)

brain stem Potassium(Minus)

Right

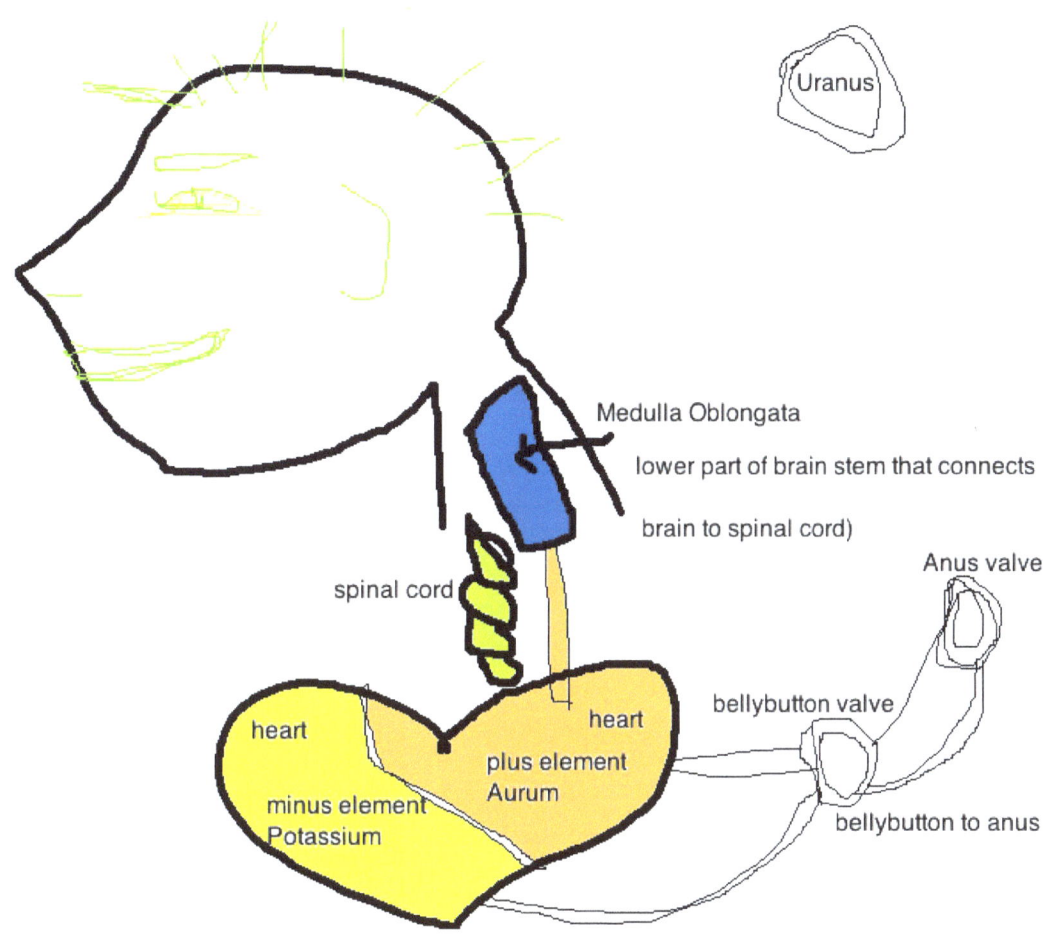

Heart:

Too much Aurum (a Plus Element): High Blood pressure, Small size heart
Discuss(A TOTALLY FICTIONAL MADE UP STORY):OK so Dick Cheney got into government
& they get lots of free steak dinners there...He was very polite so he always cleaned his plate...To
compensate for the heavy bribe gifts of steak he was forced to eat, he had to smoke cigarettes
(zinc a minus element), because artificial sweeteners(potassium a natural beta-blocker vitamin
K) weren't invented yet...But then his wife told him his smoking was stinking up the House...So
then his blood pressure skyrocketed & he had some heart attacks, due to the continuous
steaks...Plus the bribe gifters were mad because Cheney wasn't being bought because he was
pissed about the heart attacks...So doctors stepped in & put him on beta-blocker drugs to lower
his blood pressure...Potassium Vitamin K (artificial sweeteners weren't chic enough yet...) Then
he went into hyperkalemia too much potassium because the steak bringers caught on that the
steaks were killing their friend not helping him...So now he almost died of too much potassium
drugs low blood pressure...So then it was opportune for somebody to remove his heart & give
him a different heart from somebody else...Cheney's heart was all oversized & distended at this
point, from too much Potassium drugs...Low blood pressure makes your heart look real big but
really it is more flaccid, less pressure...Need I say more?
  Plus they really wanted to guinea pig someone important about how they can rip your heart
out & murder some motorcycle rider & take his heart & give it to you on a plate...The steak

gifters had an even better gift...Someone's heart on a plate...In exchange they wanted free publicity about this whole heart transplant surgery thing....Cheney wasn't buying that either...he didn't like the Kool-aid...That's why he got elected in the first place...He had a good heart...
*& that is why children should not take bribes especially if they are in government...or be forced to clean their plate if they feel full...

Heart:

 Too much Potassium (a Minus Element): Low Blood pressure, Large sizeheart, HCM HyperTrophic Cardio Myopathy (enlarged heart distended but actually missing Aurum)...
  Concussion is characterized by severely low Aurum levels & severely highPotassium levels...(There are Taurine drugs like Digitalis to add taurine/Aurum, but also please withdraw beta blocker heart potassium drugs & artificial sweeteners which contain 4 molecules of potassium if the person is in head injury state or recovering from hospital...Taurine powder can be bought at pet or human health stores & is the same stuff actually...Just mix it into a drink...)(Head injury needs to RAISE blood pressure)...(So NO potassium after head injury)...

Elements:where to find,

Heart :Aurum (a Plus Element): Gold, Taurine Powder, Clam Juice, Mussels, Nitroglycerin is a taurine drug high strength, Digitalis is a Taurine drug medium strength, Taurine is an Aurum as well but you can buy it from health supplement stores bodybuilding supplement stores & even pet supply stores as a powder(same stuff even the pet stuff humans can take too-share with your pet-hcm hypertrophicardiomyopathy is common in overbred type breeds)...Diuretics are in the Taurine category...(it also makes you pooh more)...

  Arabinogalactan is something you get from Larch trees-it is similar to Copal Amber, B12, taurine, also found in gum arabic(gum arabic is used to thicken watercolour paints if you want them to be more waterproof)...The Larch tree itself has good waterproofing abilities due to its Arabinogalactan...A new chewable chocolate flavour supplement containing this aragaloctan is called Alomune...This would be good to take if you have had a head injury & need to boost your blood pressure up...or new Concussion...Especially if the head got hit at the back of the neck area where the brain area that controls the heart is-Medulla Oblongata that brain centre is there-which is why with head injury to that back of the neck lower head area, you HAVE to treat the HEART too...

  Copal Amber beads contain Taurine & totally work if you war them against your skin...Source them from ebay or etsy-the raw ugly ones are best & freshest & get them from Lithuania cause they are just loose on the beach there...Not expensive-put one around the neck of your unconscious or comatose friend to give them extra Taurine for their heart & brain...
N Acetyl L Cysteine reacts violently with Nitroglycerin which we know is an Aurum (taurine)...Which means it is probably also a Taurine Aurum blood pressure in the heart Raiser...http://www.bodybuilding.com/fun/southfacts_cysteine.htm Oh Thank Goodness for

Clayton South...When I am in doubt & searching side effects doesn't work, then forums for side effects doesn't work, I seek out BodyBuilding guys! Yup...Lucky guess...Clayton writes that Cysteine is a Taurine precursor!(which means that it is Taurine, said fancier)...

(this is often how I figure out these long words invented by pharmaceutical companies-Google the word plus side effects...
The drugs that react with the word will be similar-if you are lucky you might recognize one of the drugs you know...

That is how you figure out what some new thing is made of...Side effects forums are handy too...

if something raised your blood pressure you could guess it's a taurine Aurum...like that!

http://breeds-dog.blogspot.com/2013/01/dilated-cardiomyopathy-in-dogs.html?m=1

Weruva Canned Cat food contains piles of Taurine Aurum...(Gold)...Makes cats purr, see better, strengthens their heart...bengals tend towards HCM (hypertrophicardiomyopathy low blood pressure so taurine is good for that)...If they start to drive you crazy though, you can throw in a cat food that has a tiny amount of potassium in it...See Potassium section below....
**Aurum is a DIURETIC (also makes one pooh)

Heart: Potassium (a Minus Element)- Artificial Sweeteners like Sweet n' low Splenda Sugar twin, Bananas, Coconut Water or Coco Juice, Yes artificial sweeteners contain potassium which lowers blood pressure(Beta blocker drugs are also potassium based) (Avoid potassium after concussion-the body needs to raise blood pressure after injury-be careful with heart drugs then-the heart can give out due to excess potassium-people who got the death penalty were killed using potassium! Really...)Note: half the salt salt contains potassium...ANTI-diuretics are in the Potassium category which includes all the bladder control type drugs...
Methionine means potassium...Menadione means potassium, sorry, these words are so long sometimes, sometimes I screw them up, sorry...
**Potassium is an ANTI-Diuretic-keeps one from peeing(also might make you swollen with liquid)...(you'd probably poop less too)...

1 Concussion & Raising Taurine levels in the Heart... - The Grove ... Jun 7, 2013 ... During & After concussion, one must try to raise Taurine levels (Aurum) in the Heart...Since Potassium is Taurine's twin opposite in the heart, ...
http://www.grovecanada.com/blog/2013/06/concussion-raising-taurine-levels-in-the-heart.html

2 Medulla Oblongata Heart Blood Pressure - The Grove Body Part ... 3 days ago ... So the Medulla Oblongata is at the bottom of the brain stem...It connects the brain to the spinal cord...From there it connects to your heart.

http://www.grovecanada.com/blog/2013/10/medulla-oblongata-heart-blood-pressure.html

3   Download 118071034-Grove-Body-Part-Chart - The Grove Body ... imbalance in a specific organ that can be corrected. *lungs & lymphs work at making muscles 12 thyroid builds bone. 8 thymus 7 makes blood heart 11 regulates.
http://www.grovecanada.com/files/118071034-grove-body-part-chart.pdf

4

B.F.F. Best feline Friend canned cat food at WOOFTOWN near summerhill LCBO in Toronto, contains some potassium...It is called Menadione on the label...Use judiciously only if you have fed too much Taurine Weruva food & the cats are driving you nuts...
You will know they are getting too much Aurum Taurine if they start to create plots like the Russians & the Afghanis did...

   You know the plot...You(Afghani guy /woman) pretend you are fighting with me, I'll)Russian guy woman) pretend I am fighting with you, & during the combat, let's kill Sari(the third party, but make it look like an accident/collateral damage)...(The Americans/Canadians/Mexicans)

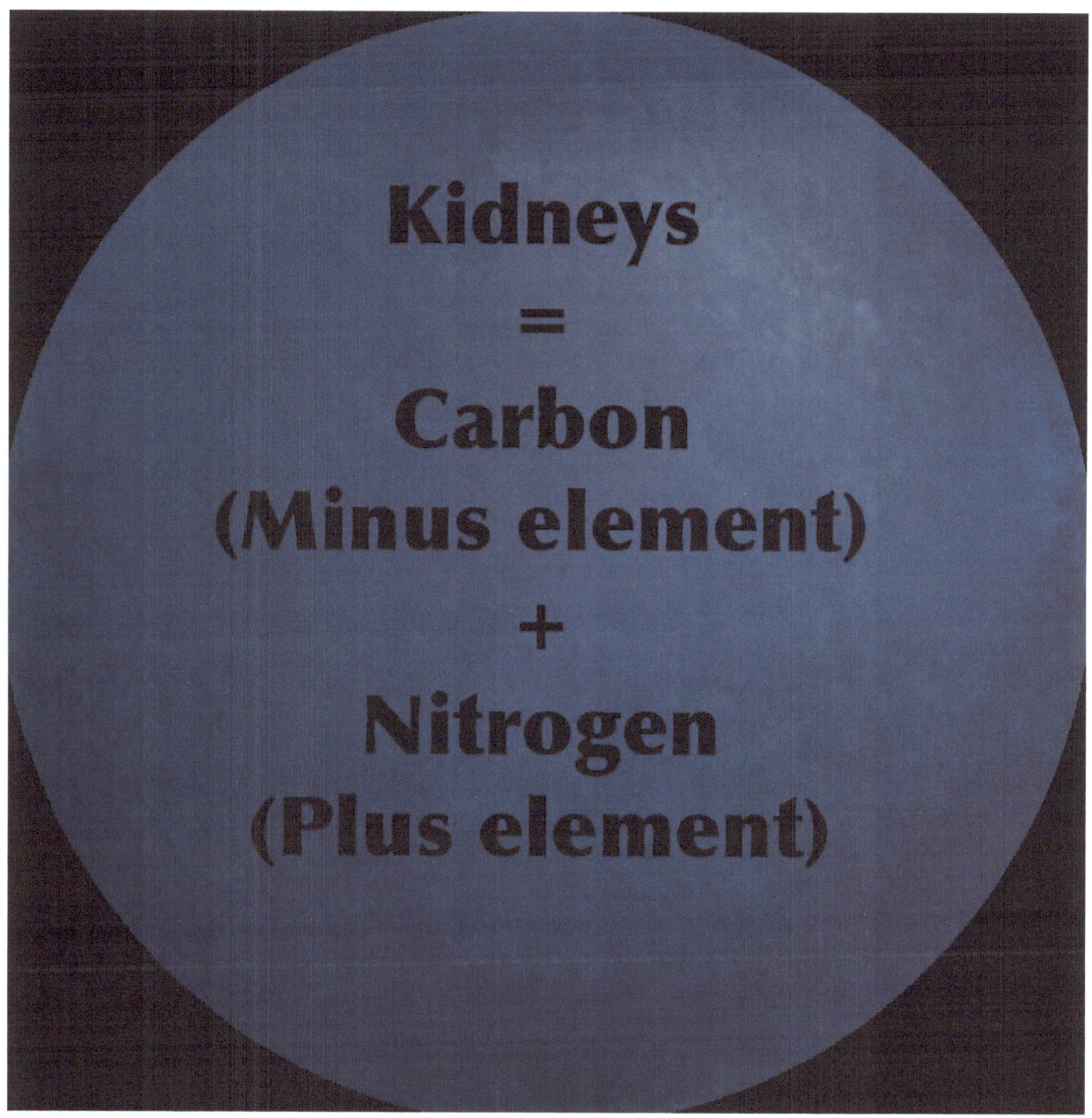

Kidneys=Carbon(Minus element)+Nitrogen(Plus element)

http://www.grovecanada.com/blog/2013/10/neurons-nerves-the-brain-stem-the-kidneys.html

Cells "renal tubes" neurons

left side of the head brain is
NITROGEN

equals right kidney right side of body
NITROGEN

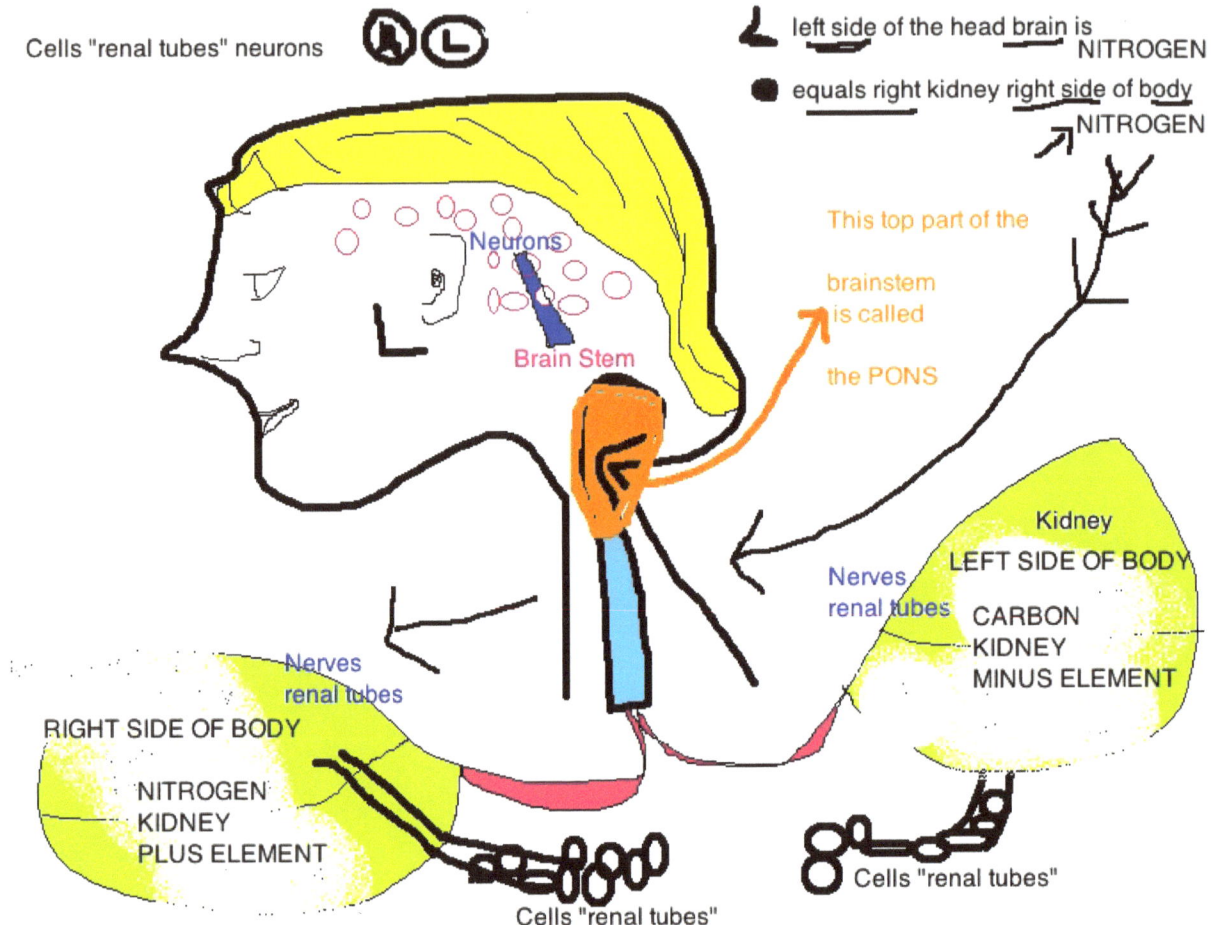

Neurons

Brain Stem

This top part of the

brainstem

is called

the PONS

Kidney
LEFT SIDE OF BODY

Nerves
renal tubes

CARBON
KIDNEY
MINUS ELEMENT

Nerves
renal tubes

RIGHT SIDE OF BODY

NITROGEN
KIDNEY
PLUS ELEMENT

Cells "renal tubes"

Cells "renal tubes"

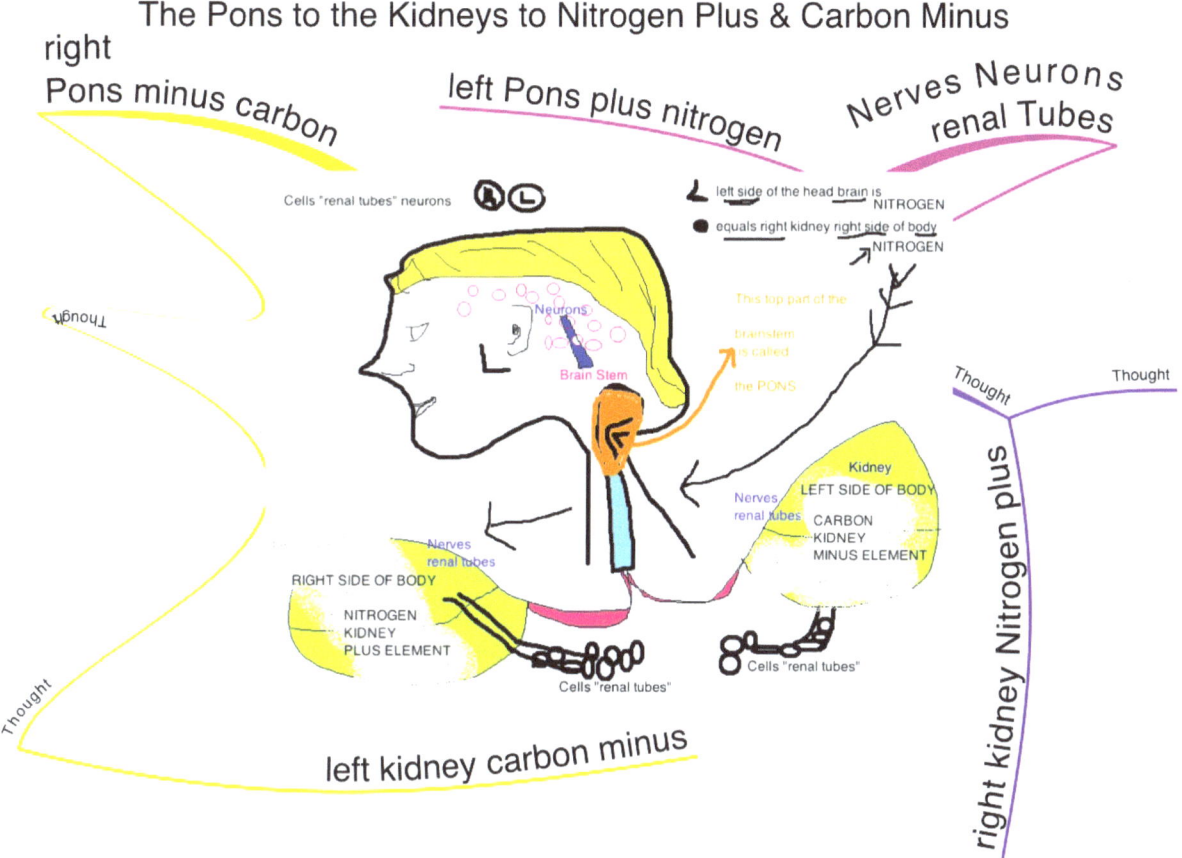

The Pons to the Kidneys to Nitrogen Plus & Carbon Minus

right Pons minus carbon

left Pons plus nitrogen

Nerves Neurons renal Tubes

left kidney carbon minus

right kidney Nitrogen plus

Kidneys:

Too much Carbon (a Minus Element):Down's Syndrome, Mongoloid appearance, low forehead, working in mechanical/cooking industry where carbon/ oil is omnipresent, Coal mining causes excess carbon...Lumber industry workers are exposed to excess CARBON...

Kidneys:

Too much Nitrogen (a Plus Element):Kidney blocks, Kidney failures, need for Dialysis...Excess Nitrogen (in athletic supplements that enhance performance can also create a severe type of depression which manifests as homicidal tendencies or extreme aggressiveness to others)....Hateful...Aggressive...Dislike of others...
Coeliac or Celiac disease is too much Nitrogen...

http://www.best-gout-remedies.com/bakingsoda.html After much deliberation & false steps, I have decided to put Gout into the Nitrogen excess category of the Kidneys...Why? Ok, because uric acid is high in Gout sufferers & that is a Nitrogen predominant thing...Also, because when you eat too many Nitrogen things, you can get a kidney blockage type thing, which manifests as pain in your big toe on the right hand side...I have noticed Gout sufferers lean towards the right

big toe...(left big toe usually indicates a more serious heart involvement, it can indicate a Nitrogen excess too, but on the left side it is a more serious problem...-) For example, you eat a fast food pizza made with a genetically modified GMO grain pizza crust...Half an hour later you get a severe cramp in your right foot...I see Gout as being a more chronic form of this...Ok next reason why I think Gout is a Nitrogen excess...Because there is an 85% recovery rate when Gout sufferers take baking soda(with some water, like a tablespoon...see the link above..) Baking soda is sodium bicarbonate which means really it is a Carbon...Carbon is like in oil, like olive oil...Carbon is opposite to Nitrogen in the Kidneys...The fact that Carbon works for Gout says to me that Gout is a Nitrogen excess problem...So that is my argument for Gout...Apologies for all my false steps on this one...This was actually pretty hard to figure out...!!!
***So...There is a strong correlation between Gout & Celiac & Gluten intolerance...So cutting back on all glutens will help Gout enormously...Or switch to eating ONLY organic glutens which clears out all Genetically Modified Organisms which get stuck in your Kidneys...Many people think they are Celiac Or Gout-y, only to discover their problem is only with GMO glutens & grains, that organic grains go through with no problem!(Drinking a little olive oil or canola oil or safflower oil, daily, helps ensure any GMO grains you do eat don't get stuck!)...Another tried & true remedy for Gout is Coconut oil, 1 tablespoon 3 times a day...The Carbon in the Coconut oil gets rid of the Nitrogen uric acid buildup well...

Fri. Jan 3, 2014: before dinner at Dynasty (great Yorkville Chinese food), I mentioned to Joseph about how I see Gout as a Nitrogen excess, but how many doctors refer to Gout as an "arthritis" which I don't really see...Anyways, he told me that his (non-biological) brother Carl had gout...Which I said was very very unusual for someone with Down's Syndrome, because Down's is a carbon excess, & Gout is a Nitrogen excess, & carbon & Nitrogen are Opposites in the Kidneys...Meaning that if Carl had now a Nitrogen excess, that somehow his Down's had been corrected over time...After dinner (delicious by the way), I checked...Yup...Yes...Gout is incredibly incredibly rare in Down's Syndrome...because, as I mentioned, Nitrogen & Carbon are opposites...It would be like saying your anorexic friend was now obese...Very unusual...Here's a study http://www.ncbi.nlm.nih.gov/pmc/articles/PMC1010266/pdf/annrheumd00354-0067.pdf (they found only 6 subjects with Down's who also had Gout...)(They talk about the scarcity of this phenomenon...They should read this book to understand the why! Big smile)!

The actor William Shatner sold one of his Kidney stones on Ebay for 75 thousand dollars...On a recent roast(those vile comedy shows where people insult each other for money), Shatner explained that his Kidney stone was made of Uric acid(Nitrogen) & Calcium combined...This is useful to know, because then, theoretically, one could dissolve or prevent a kidney stone by adding both Carbon & Iodine to one's diet...(Carbon & Iodine are opposites to Nitrogen & Calcium)...

Elements:where to find,

Kidneys: Nitrogen (a Plus Element):Tea Tree Oil, Eucalyptus Leaves, Leafs, Chlorophyll containing Green Things, Clorets, Essential Oil Eucalyptus, Barley

Grass Powder, Arginine Powder is a great source of Nitrogen & is easy to find at BodyBuilding Supplement stores like Popeye's in Toronto(this definitely works from neuron regrowth-put a tiny amount into lemon juice & water & drink-it is sourced from BEETS), Wheatgrass Juice, Salads, More esoteric source(& more $$) is Lion's Mane Mushroom Extract for Nitrogen (mushrooms are grown in Nitrogen to make them bigger...)Nitrogen is also called Beta- Alanine in bodybuilding supplements...Nitrogen makes one smarter- like for Down's Syndrome applications...But Nitrogen can also cause urinary tract
infections, so be careful...Also Nitrogen can make one hateful to others...(athletes often take Nitrogen for stamina, girth & smarts- but it also makes them so mean!)
Phenylalanine means Nitrogen(lord let's put a halt on all new words!)
Ammonium carbonate is a Nitrogen dominant thing also called Smelling Salts...(It also contains some carbon is dioxide form which just means gaseous form)...You use smelling slats when someone has fainted to wake them up...The Nitrogen gives them energy...To the kidneys...
Miso, like found in Miso soup, is a bean ground into a powder, or a barley, a grain, so it falls into the Nitrogen category of elements(girth builder, smarts builder, stamina builder but also can cause hateful personality & UTIs urinary tract infections)...
*Rust en Vrede red wine from South Africa, a shiraz, seems to contain alot of Nitrogen...It was around $25 Cad at the LCBO recently)...(How did I know? A couple of sips & I became aggressive...Nitrogen things do that to you...Which is why people in bars tend to be ruder...)
*Those white Mexican (large) Kidney Beans seem to contain a high amount of Nitrogen, based on the combination of high energy on a wintry day & aggressive rudeness I experienced after eating two bean wraps prior...It seems I can't get my Nitrogen energy veggies without getting ruder, maybe I need to throw in some cautionary olive oil to ensure I stay nice while eating my vegetables!

Carbon (a Minus Element): Oil, Olive oil, Fish Oil, Hair Conditioner, Suntan Oil, Coconut Oil, Canola Oil, Corn Oil, Coal Mining, Greasy things (exhaust from cars, planes, boats, will also contain carbon) (working in a restaurant exposes one to carbon, oils), Butter & margarine contain carbon too...(Carbon makes one nicer, kinder, but can also cause IQ loss)...
*Neat trick:Take a swig (a chug) daily, or once in a while, of oil, like canola oil or corn oil or olive oil or safflower oil, to alleviate the blocked feeling you get from GMO glutens or your Celiac problem...(in about 24 hours you pooh out the block)...

Yes, Carbon dioxide the exhaust from cars falls into the Carbon...

Leaded Gasoline from boats contains both Carbon & Lead...There was a boat at Bluffer's Park this summer of 2013 that was using Leaded gasoline...The Lead made my left toenail look ugly (thick & fungussy)...

Alka Seltzer contains Baking soda(Sodium bicarbonate which is Carbon plus sodium, salt), plus, Titanium(Aspirin)...Alka Seltzer works for Gout, though because of the Titanium(aspirin) be aware too much can cause memory loss...

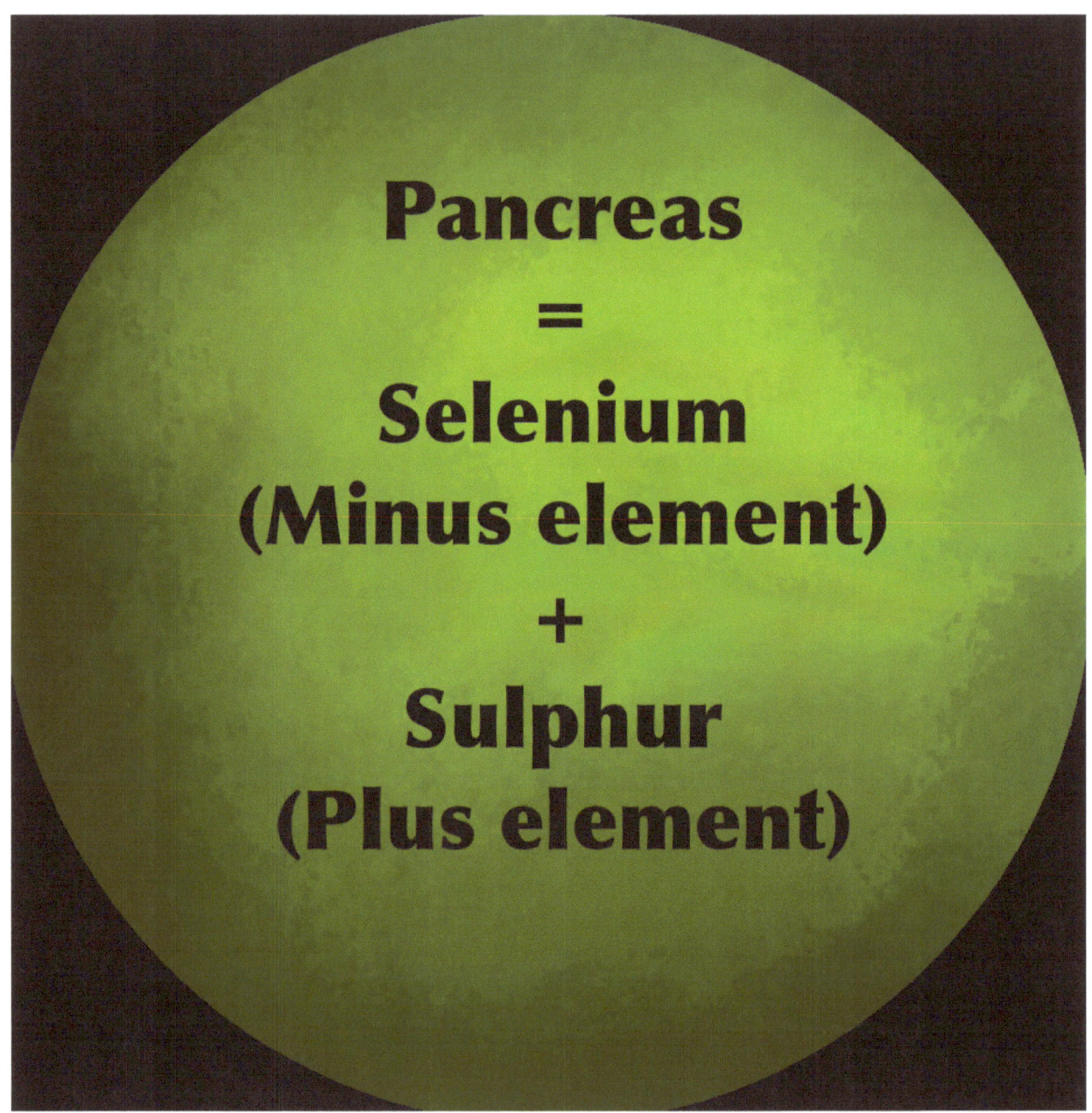

Pancreas=Selenium(Minus element)+Sulphur(Plus element)

Eyes to Occipital Lobe to Pancreas to Selenium Minus & Sulphur Plus

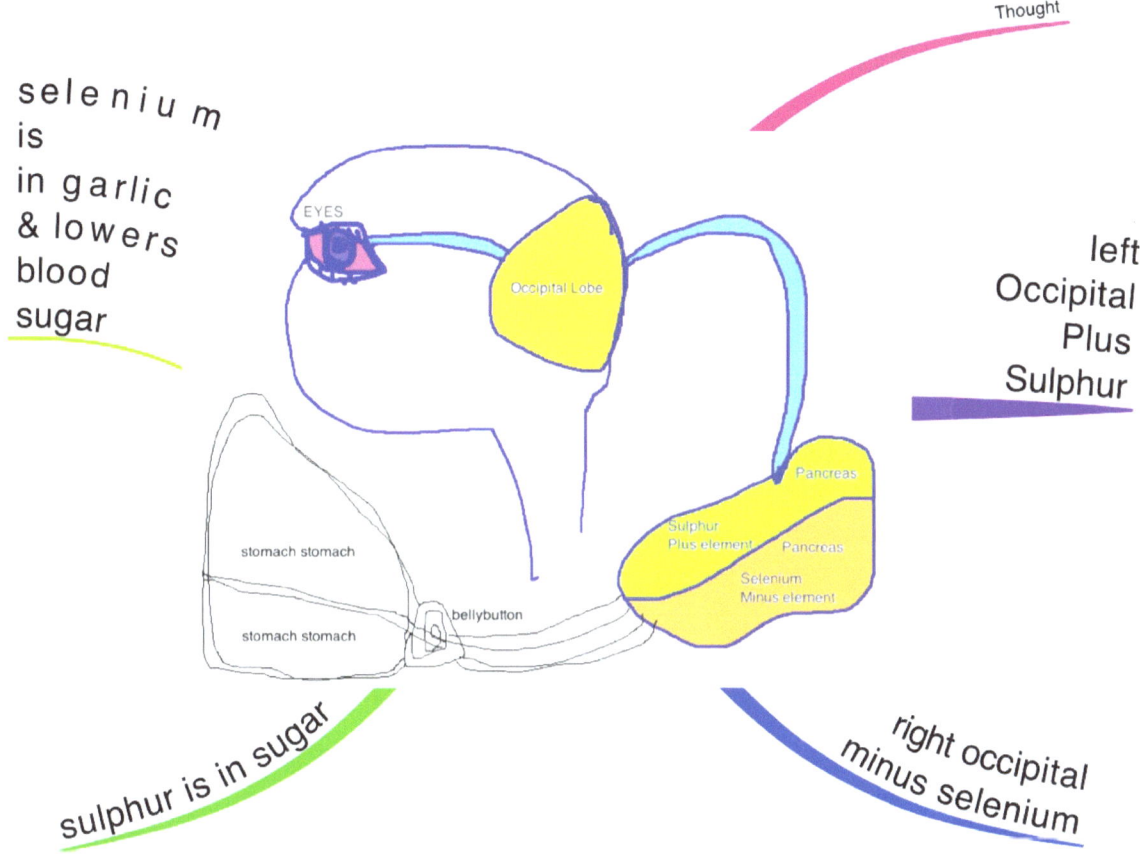

selenium
is
in garlic
& lowers
blood
sugar

Thought

left
Occipital
Plus
Sulphur

sulphur is in sugar

right occipital
minus selenium

http://www.grovecanada.com/blog/2013/10/eyes-occipital-lobe-pancreas.html

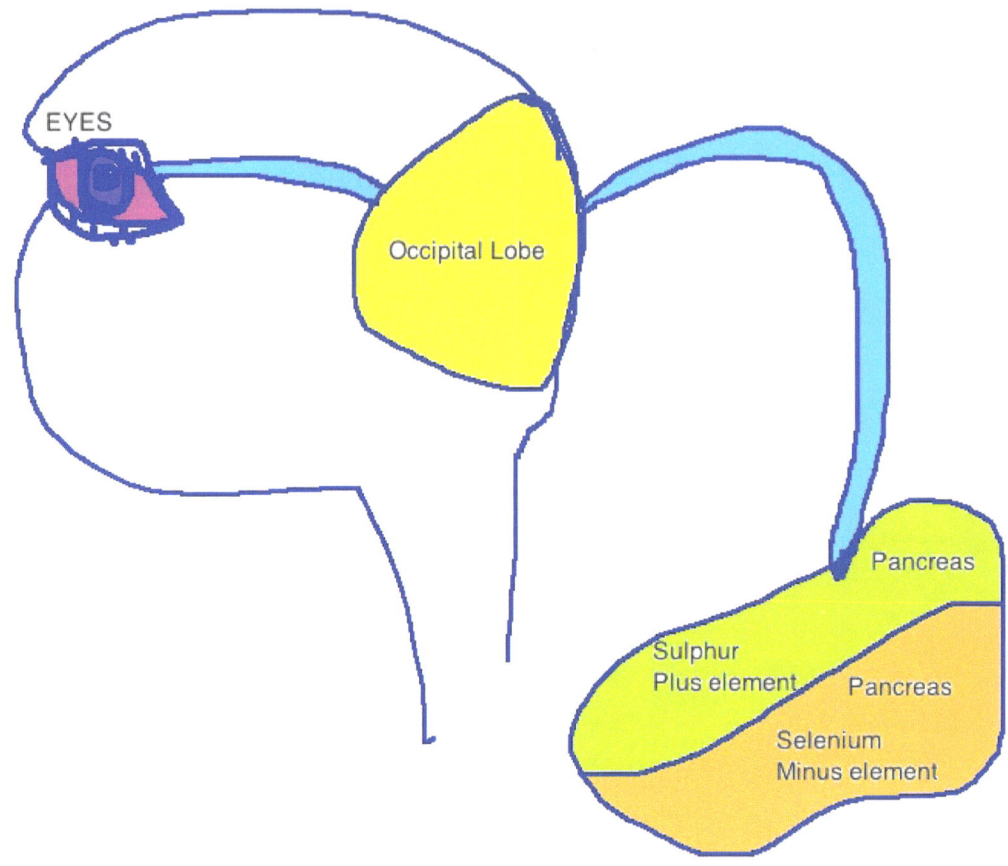

Pancreas:

Too much Selenium (a Minus Element): bad breath,dizzy spells, coma, low blood sugar

Pancreas:

Too much Sulphur (a Plus Element): Diabetes, Herpes, Dandruff, shingles, pimples, rotten painful teeth & gums...Glaucoma, macular degeneration, cataracts-high blood sugar related...Diabetic retinopathy...Eye problems related to high blood sugar/sulphur ...Psoriasis is also excess Sulphur(Sugars)...

1 Download 118071034-Grove-Body-Part-Chart - The Grove Body ... Sulphur is found in Sugar, & can cause Diabetes in excess dose. ... Fruit by the way contains plenty of sugar, so if you are diabetic, don't pig out on fruit either.
http://www.grovecanada.com/files/118071034-grove-body-part-chart.pdf

2 Update on fixing Cartilage Degeneration, Rheumatoid Arthritis, Back ... Nov 22, 2012 ... Sadistic sulphuric acid Sade Marquis de sugars diabetic ... *p.s. Blindness due to Diabetes is because sugar is from the element SULPHUR S ...

http://www.grovecanada.com/blog/2012/11/update-on-fixing-cartilage-degeneration-rheumatoid-arthritis-back-pains-due-to-slipped-discs-that-so.html

3   The Grove Body Part Chart...: August 2012 Aug 26, 2012... to lower the blood sugar/ sulfur in the pancreas if you are afraid or are already of being diabetic...This is completely unrelated to points 1), 2), ...
http://www.grovecanada.com/blog/2012/08/page/2/

Elements:where to find,

 Pancreas,
Selenium (a Minus Element): Garlic, Garlic Capsules, Antibiotics, Insulin, Tonic Water (quinine)

Sulphur (a Plus Element): Sugar, sugars, Turpentine,Some expensive hair conditioners contain sulphur sugar...

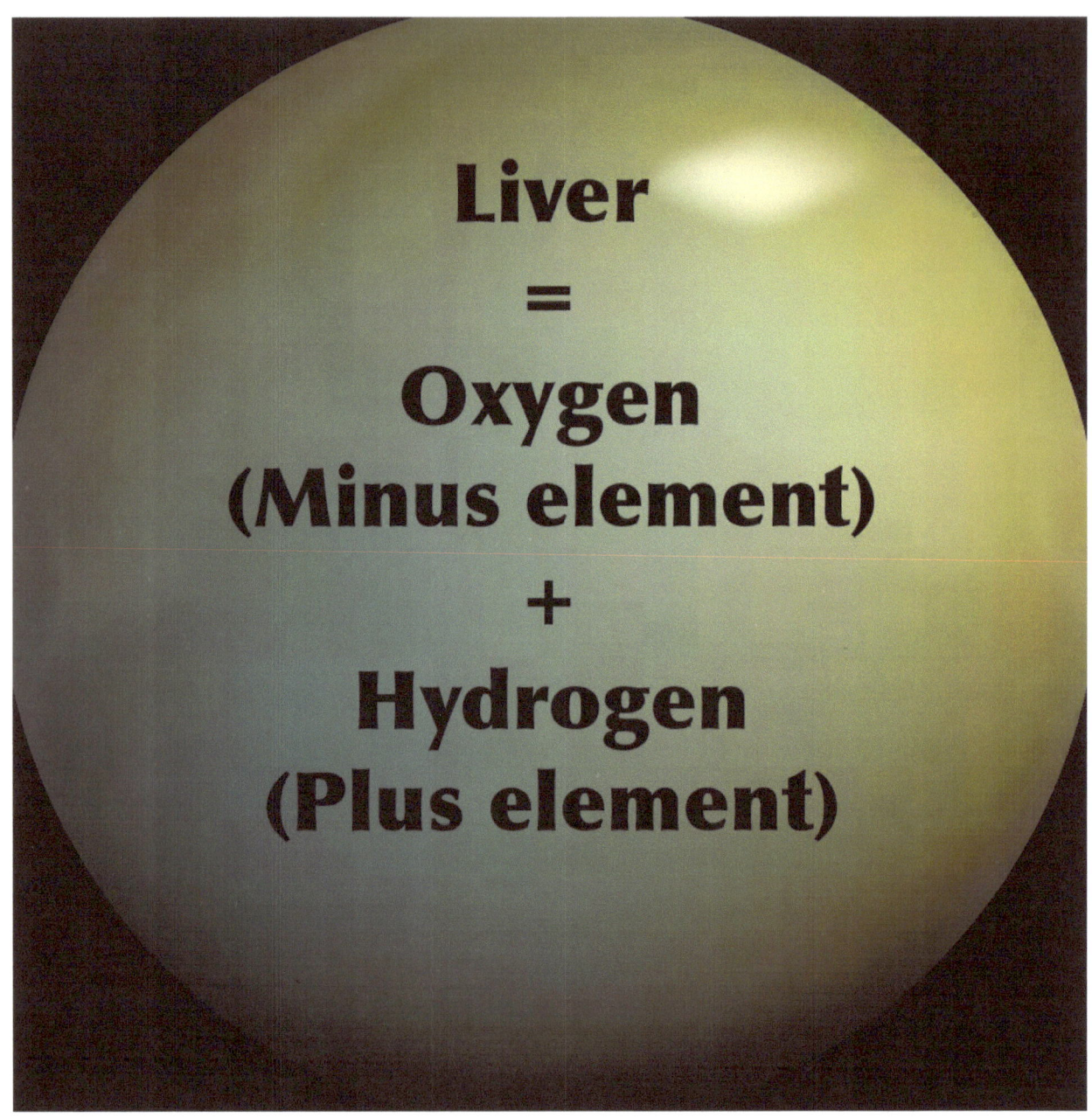

Liver=Oxygen(Minus element)+Hydrogen(Plus element)

http://www.grovecanada.com/blog/2013/10/cerebellum-liver-hydration.html

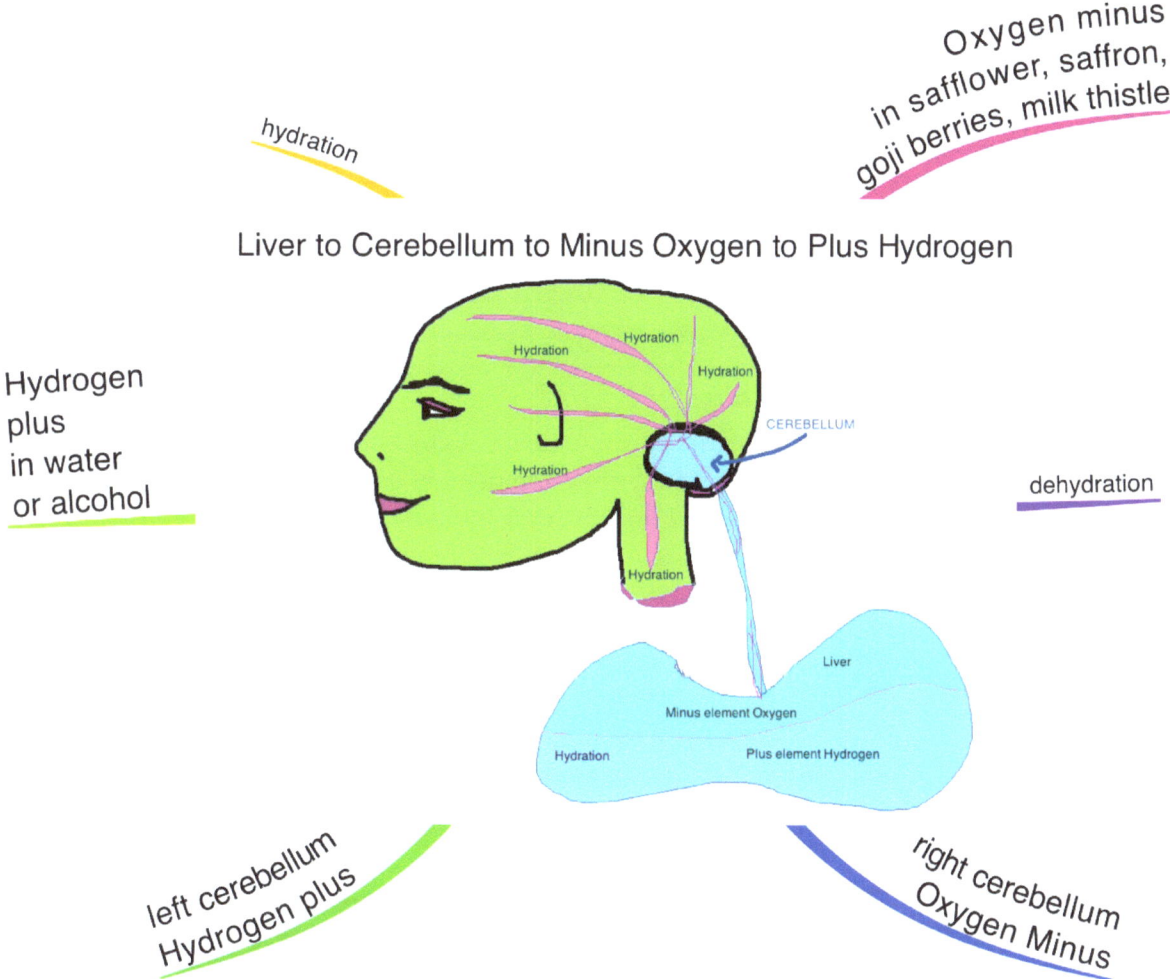

Liver: (euvolemia means a normal fluid balance in the body...Not too much water, not too much oxygen, A Goldilocks amount! That's euvolemia)...Ok technically euvolumia refers to how much blood volume is in the body...But water hydrogen oxygen air levels affect blood volume...So by watching both your water & oxygen intake, you can alter your blood volume...up or down...

Too much Oxygen (a Minus Element): dehydration, dry mouth

Liver:

Too much Hydrogen (a Plus Element): Hepatitis(holes in liver allow water to get in), Common Cold, Chronic Fatigue Syndrome, Epstein Barr disease, Hydrocephalic (water on brain)...Excess Hydrogen can also cause depression-this type of depression is inward & can lead to suicidal tendencies...

Myalgic Encephalomyelitis, ME(Just another name for a similar thing-a question of degree), mononuceosis (Mono)...Migraines...

http://www.ehow.com/info_8095135_rashes-skin-associated-colds.html

  Sari's Note:However, on second thought, I remember my across the street neighbour having Calamine lotion fights with her brother when the family all had chicken pox together...Calamine is a selenium based thing which clears up & soothes the chicken pox spots...Since calamine is a Selenium element, & Sulphur(think Sugar) is its opposite, I'd correct myself & say that, really, measles, rubella, & chicken pox, are primarily SULPHUR excess imbalances, with the Hydrogen excess being only a secondary excess...Which makes sense because the Pancreas comes before the Liver in our list & in the body...So the cold type symptoms you might get, are just secondary Hydrogen excess, not primary cause imbalance...Thus, really, one should pull away from Sulphurs(sugars) in measles, chicken pox & rubella...

Hydrocephalism is water on the brain-Yup Hydrogen excess...(The words "brain fog" might describe water on the brain in a hot place so you are actually getting STEAM in the brain causing a brain fog, literally!

*which is described as a "brain fog")

Hepatic Encephalopathy, Hydrocephaly-this just means water on the brain, hepatic is liver, hydro is water(solution is to dry out or dehydrate the person, administering Oxygen can help with this as well as pulling away from all liquids(hydrogens)Translation-dehydrate the body & brain if the person is drowning or hydrocephalic(times when water is really really really the wrong thing to give!!!)...

**chronic traumatic encephalopathy-getting hit in the head many many times...often causes water on the brain in the damaged areas, so Hydrogen excess...EDEMA of the brain(swelling with liquid parts)

 **"punch-drunk" syndrome in boxers and prizefighters before the 1930s.(they act like drunk people, hydrogen excess, 'cause of the extra water hydrogen on the brain from getting hit so much there...

***Comment about self-medicating: Sometimes severe back pain can cause a person to self-medicate with alcohol...So we have a Magnesium excess(the pain) causing someone to self-medicate with Hydrogen(alcohol)...The Hydrogen excess can cause suicidal tendencies...Depression...Now the person has depression...But maybe cured the back pain since Hydrogen will break down to Mercury another Plus element, over time...But now they are depressed...They stop drinking & the back pain comes back...Go figure...Anyways, be careful when self-medicating...KNOW WHEN TO STOP...KNOW WHAT AMOUNT CURES YOU & WHAT AMOUNT TIPS YOU OVER THE EDGE INTO A NEW DISEASE...

**so...sometimes people who have acid reflux, a copper excess, will drink too much water, Hydrogen...Then they get something like CFS due to too much water drinking...But the original problem is the copper excess...They are self-medicating with water, Hydrogen...A better solution for acid reflux, copper excess, is Phosphorus...L' tryptophan is a Phosphorus thing...Like hot turkey or warmed milk or old cheese...(mold is also Phosphorus so be careful)...

**some people will have fibromyalgia, a magnesium excess, so they self-medicate with alcohol, another Hydrogen but heavier...Then they get liver related (wetness, hydrogen excess) problems...A better solution for magnesium excess is mercury...Like go live near a volcano... (active ones spew cartilage building Mercury, but even inactive ones, the rock is rich with Mercury)...An active volcano can be hazardous to your health as a by the way... :)

Varicose veins seem to get either better or worse depending on Hydrogen & Oxygen balance...More Hydrogen, worse...More Oxygen, better...Saffron is a great Oxygen source, especially if you eat it straight as a powder or chew the threads without cooking it...(tastes bitter)!

***are you depressed? Stop drinking 8 glasses of water a day...Hydrogen excess causes depression...The first thing you need to do is back away from your water addiction!

Factoid: (from)2009 — "One quarter of patients with chronic tooth pain, jaw/face pain, or arthritis use alcohol for pain relief." (my comment:which can lead to a secondary problem, called Depression due to the Hydrogen excess...So be careful! Don't Over-self-medicate!)

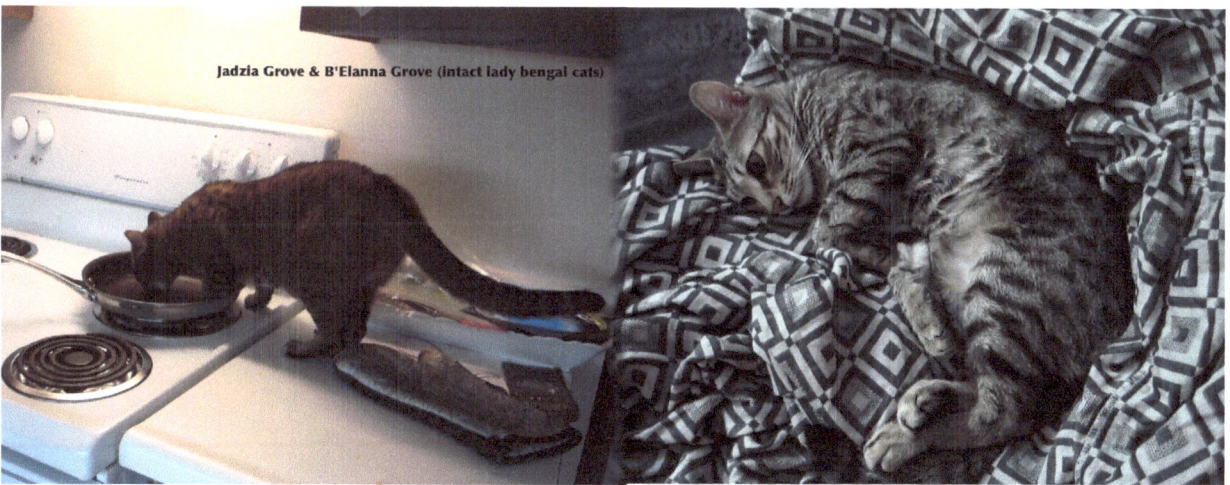

Jadzia Grove & B'Elanna Grove (intact lady bengal cats)

(I feel it is time for a picture of cats! These are GroveCanada cats!)...(Jadzia born April 16, 2005 snow gold, B'Elanna born Dec. 1st, 2004 snow silver)

(In response to the question:Is she sweet?): "Hmm...Ok so Joseph would say :"Why? Do you want her?"...Hmm...In the world of comedy, cats are king...Within the Kings, bengal cats are like the lead protagonist in anything that is funny...They will drop things off your counter just to watch them fall...They consistently seek out the funniest positions, words, behaviours, just to get a laugh...They are also very wild...They are cat but to all the extremes...To this day, when Joseph approaches B'Elanna her ears throw back & she growls like a bloodthirsty animal...She loves him too...Her paw can slash at you faster than any Southpaw boxer, & you will find yourself hemorrhaging from a crucial artery...But is she sweet? Yes...She purrs so loud it drowns out the tv set as she sits on my lap...They both talk...My mum had a conniption when B'Elanna said:"Hi" when she was just out of being a kitten...She is happy to have a bath, can play fetch (those charity bracelets made of silicone do well), has her ovaries, can speak & does, & is very good with the computer...With ovaries, they cost about 2 grand, which was why we didn't get a new car for many years-we chose expensive cats instead...(I did get a breeder's licence & various things so we could keep them intact without getting into arguments with Bob Barker)! p.s.. I think she loves you, she came over to sit on my lap while I am typing...She turned 9 on December 1st & has been feeling vulnerable about it..."

Each Organ has 2 Opposing Elements...(Minus & Plus)

Organ	Minus Element	Plus Element
Thyroid	Zinc	Lead
Thymus	Manganese	Iron
Lungs & Lymph Nodes	Titanium	Aluminum
Heart	Potassium	Aurum
Kidneys	Carbon	Nitrogen
Pancreas	Selenium	Sulphur
Liver	Oxygen	Hydrogen
Adrenal Gland	Iodine	Calcium
Spleen	Copper	Phosphorus
Gallbladder	Magnesium	Mercury
Colon	Fluorine	Bismuth

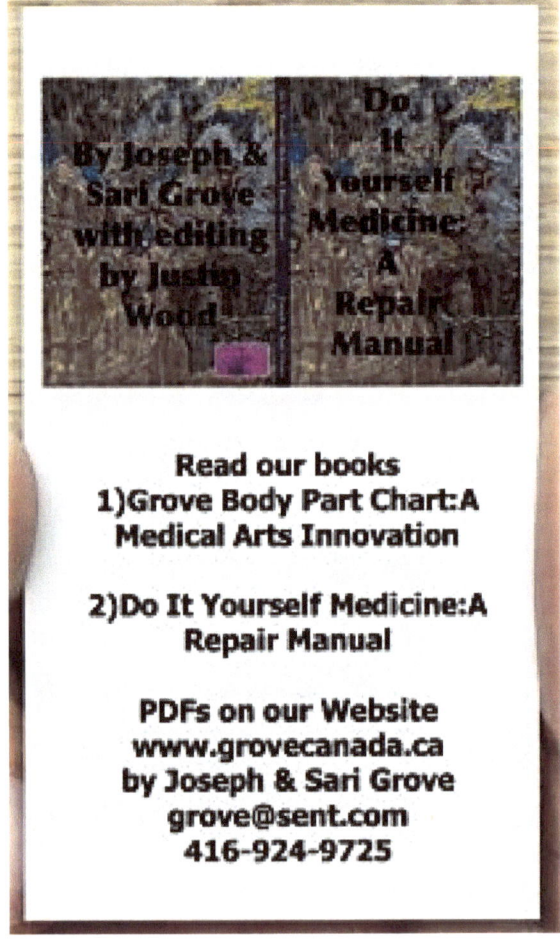

By Joseph & Sari Grove with editing by Justin Wood

Do It Yourself Medicine: A Repair Manual

Read our books
1)Grove Body Part Chart:A Medical Arts Innovation

2)Do It Yourself Medicine:A Repair Manual

PDFs on our Website www.grovecanada.ca by Joseph & Sari Grove grove@sent.com 416-924-9725

Elements:where to find,

Liver: Oxygen (a Minus Element): Goji berries, Milk Thistle, Dandelion Greens, Fresh Clean Air, Lycopene is Oxygen, Lycopene is found in Tomatoes & in the green part of tomato like the leafs & stem too
http://www.google.nl/patents/WO2000078325A1?cl=en

Oxygen is in(can be found in) Hydrogen PERoxide (a wet Oxygen like Perrier water or OZONated water)!

*Strawberry & Strawberry leaf are more Oxygen elements(words like tannin or atropine or cyanide indicate Oxygen)...The raspberry itself is an Oxygen, but the leaf of the raspberry is much more of an Iodine element see Adrenal Gland...My favorite source of Oxygen is GOJI berries because you can eat them...

http://www.ncbi.nlm.nih.gov/pmc/articles/PMC3003214/ *Grape seeds & Grape seed extract are also an OXYGEN substance...The study just shows how grape seed extract can reverse or prevent cirrhosis(my words, just summing up)...

  (i'd also use grape seeds, proanthocyanidins is another word for Oxygen btw, to treat the common cold & Chronic fatigue syndrome, & hepatitis-all liver things characterized by Hydrogen excess thus needing Oxygen elements...)

http://www.healwithfood.org/health-benefits/whole-grape-seeds-edible.php Eating the seeds of grapes, you chew them, has all sorts of benefits like anti-depressant, drying up varicose veins, weight loss, anti-common cold...

There is an herbal pill called Flavay which is a combo of Titanium & Oxygen...(pine bark & grape seeds)...That would be good for someone with asthma & the common cold together...Since asthma is an aluminum excess & the common cold is a hydrogen excess... (***note:Not a huge fan of combo pills, since they have to be so precise-it's like a long recipe-what if you are allergic to pineapple? or nuts?Now the whole meal cannot be eaten...)

The Autumn Crocus(which has been made into a drug called Colchicine), also known as Meadow saffron(this stuff is stronger than the stuff you know & is regulated), Regular Saffron(contains the same stuff as the drug one, but like less)-are things that contain large amounts of Oxygen...

  (***The drug comes from the root of the autumn crocus, the saffron food comes from the stamens or stigmas(the red skinny things in the middle of the flower) of another Crocus flower-though both provide Oxygen to the Liver, just more or less...Regular saffron can be poisonous too at 5 grams or more)...(Quick thought:You can chew about 6 stigmas of Saffron at a time to get the Oxygen medicinal effect that cleans out a wet liver...There is a business method called "Six Sigma"-one wonders if it came from Six Stigmas originally!)

Overdose resembles arsenic overdose, which is also an Oxygen thing..Studies with Saffron have shown it for sure cleans out a Hydrogen wet soaked Liver...Confirmation it is an Oxygen element...(um, you can get Saffron powder on Amazon.com & I got like 5 grams for something like $37 dollars which is a steal deal-so, you can just take a teeny tiny thimbleful, like a thumbelina thimble, & just stick that in your mouth & eat that straight of the ground regular saffron powder, & that will give you a hit of Oxygen fast-for people catching a cold or getting rid of a cold or people with wet livers or CFS chronic fatigue syndrome-this is a good one!!!)

Cost thought:Ok so Saffron is full of Oxygen but it is also expensive...So...There is an alternative...Today I found for $3.99 about 8 grams of Organic SAFFLOWER, which is a common (much cheaper)substitute for Saffron...Safflower comes in a clear box too, & you can eat it straight from the box & it tastes like hay...Safflower is also an Oxygen element...If you have a runny nose or cold or worse, just eat the dry safflower straight...Cut back on all liquids & in a few hours, you will feel your nose dry up...It works!

Oxygen Elements continued:EGGPLANT...(the Nightshade family of vegetables, ok some say tomato is a fruit, but anyways, they all contain varying amounts of Oxygen...Eggplant more...) ****Also, did you know the seeds of an apple contain arsenic? Arsenic is an OXYGEN family thing, just way way stronger! (I know what you're thinking, could I eat apple seeds Oxygen to cure my CFS chronic fatigue syndrome? Let me doublecheck that neat idea!
http://www.rawpaleodietforum.com/omnivorous-raw-paleo/what-is-the-issue-with-nightshades/ (eggplant mmm fried, mmm Oxygen) excerpt from that link:"fried eggplants are truly delicious, home made tomato catchup or just onion and tomato salad simply delicious!" Sari's comment:YUMMY!

http://organiceyourlife.com/b-17-eat-your-apple-seeds/ eat your apple seeds(Oxygen, cyanide, arsenic!)

I'd like to reiterate if I have not already that fresh ripe cherries are an OXYGEN element...Um delicious too! (we had some from Chile which were mm mm good)...

http://www.ncbi.nlm.nih.gov/pmc/articles/PMC3003214/ This link is about grape seeds...How they clean out a wet liver...You can chew grape seeds...Grape seeds contain OXYGEN...They say they absorb better if you chew grape seeds rather than swallowing them whole...I guess you could crush them with a mortar & pestle & sprinkle the powder into your cereal or on your salad...You can also split open grape seed capsules to get the same thing & spend more money...

Mandarin Orange Peels: Are full of Oxygen...Eat your citrus(oranges, graperuits, mandarins, tangerines, lemons) peels to get Oxygen to clean out your wet liver!!! (probably the least expensive way to get Oxygen to your Liver fast!)...

Oxygen afterthoughts: I like the organic safflower the best...It's cheap, you eat it straight from the container, it tastes ok, & works quickly if you have a runny nose or are catching a cold...(It's also labelled American saffron sometimes...) Great liver cleanser...

Orris root powder is the root powder of the Iris flower...You can buy Orris root powder pretty much anywhere...This is a strong OXYGEN element...

Oxygen elements can have diarrhea as a side effect & in women can induce their period early...But they are great for curing the common cold, curing chronic fatigue syndrome, & any other task that requires cleaning & drying out a wet liver...

Another Oxygen is dried Mulberries...They are sweet, like raisins with a slight nuttiness...I got a bag from Whole Foods market yesterday...Not hard to find...(though $14.99)...

I got 5 grams of real Saffron powder from Amazon...Saffron is a powerful Oxygen, but the powder is bitter...I took a bit on the end of my knife...I can get husband to eat the Safflower, but I fear the Saffron powder will be too bitter to get him to try more than once...(a wise person once said:"Herbs don't work if you don't take them"...)

Liver: Hydrogen (a Plus Element)-Water, Alcohol, Liquids *generally, Glue
http://www.undergroundhealth.com/23-seniors-died-after-receiving-this-years-flu-shot-sold-by-pharmacies/ The flu shot can make you get the flu, as you probably already know...I got one, got sick(with the flu), that was the end of flu shots in our house...Flu, pneumonia is Hydrogen excess by the way...(swine flu is different-see gallbladder Page)

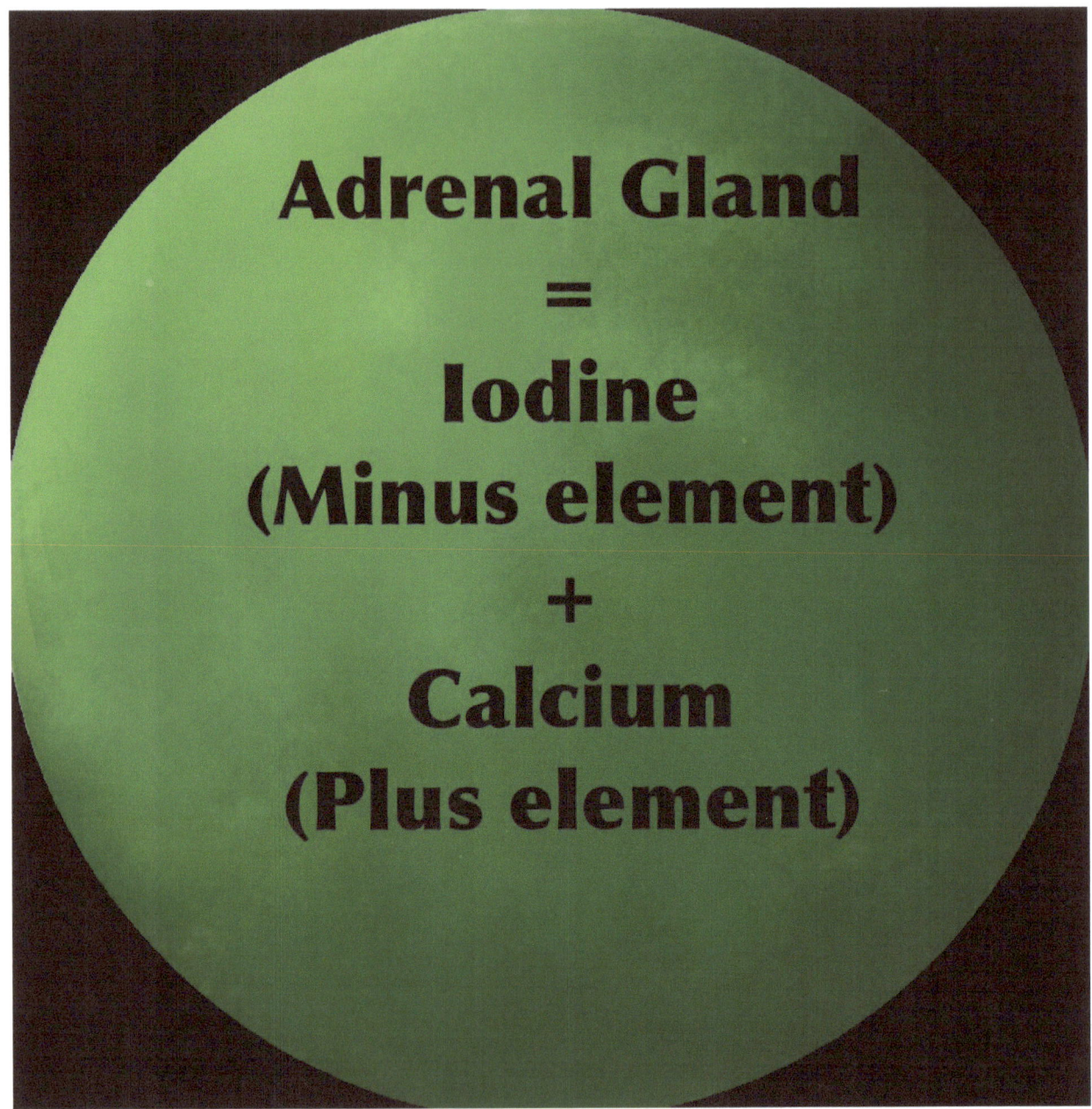

Adrenal Gland=Iodine(Minus element)+Calcium(Plus element)

left pituitary side plus calcium

Pituitary Gland to Adrenal Gland to Calcium Plus to Iodine Minus

Iodine Minus on left side of body

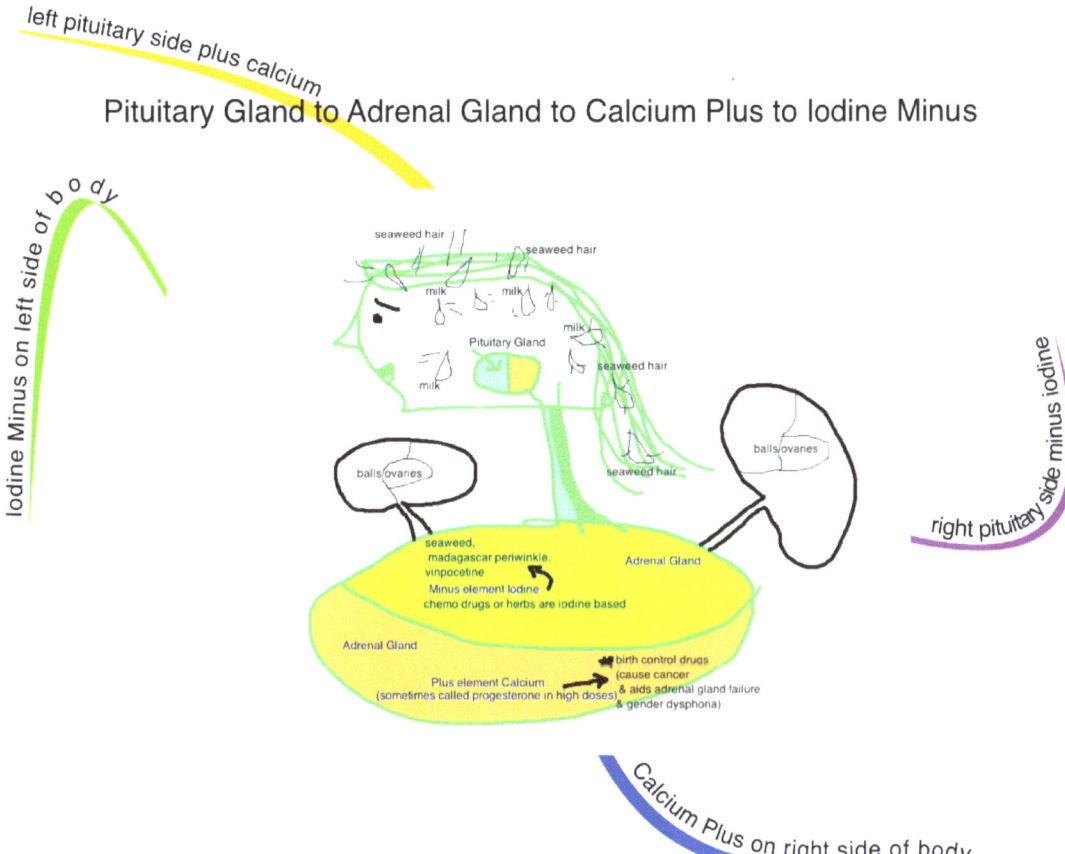

seaweed hair

seaweed hair

milk   milk

Pituitary Gland

milk

milk

seaweed hair

milk

balls/ovaries

balls/ovaries

seaweed hair

right pituitary side minus iodine

seaweed,
madagascar periwinkle,
vinpocetine

Minus element Iodine
chemo drugs or herbs are iodine based

Adrenal Gland

Adrenal Gland

Plus element Calcium
(sometimes called progesterone in high doses)

birth control drugs
(cause cancer
& aids adrenal gland failure
& gender dysphoria)

Calcium Plus on right side of body

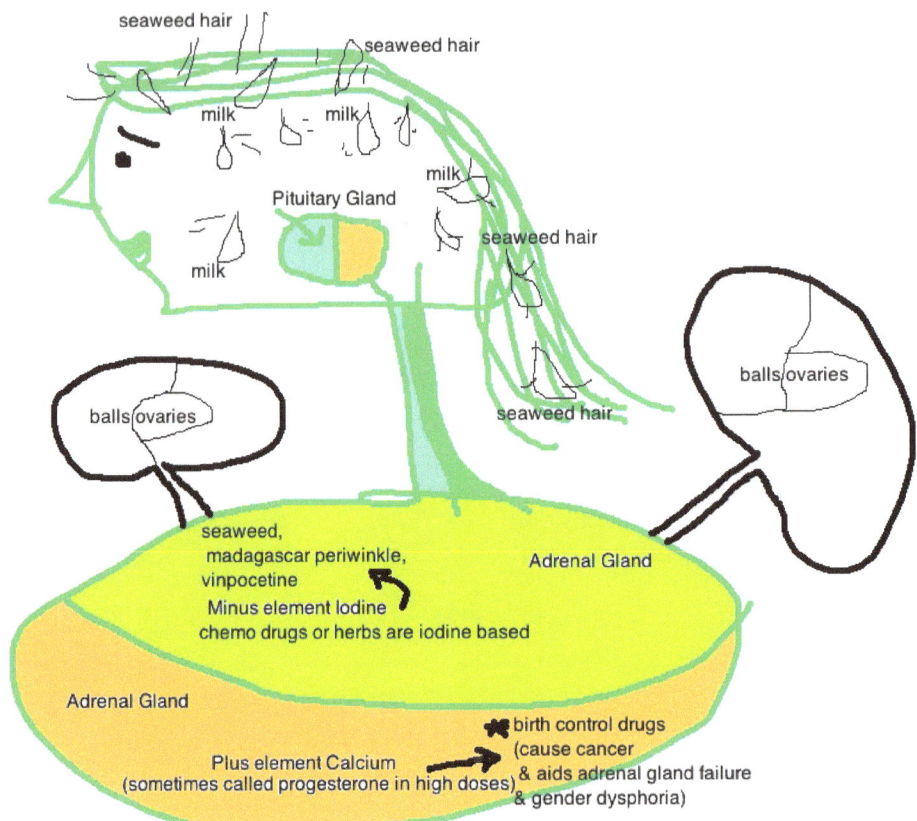

Adrenal Gland:

Too much Iodine (a Minus Element): Grave's disease, Bulging Eyes, Skinny- ness,Early Menopause, Shorter Menstrual Cycle, Bleedy, Dementia, Hemophilia, Dementia(excess warfarin is excess iodine & causes bleedy-ness
which affects thinking & cognition)...Addison's disease(John F. kennedy had this) is too much Iodine...

Adrenal Gland:

 Too much Calcium (a Plus Element):Progesterone heavy Calcium deposits mimicking Cancerous Tumours, Cancer, Lumps, Varicose veins, AIDS (which is just adrenal gland failure), gender dysphoria(ie:"dude looks like a lady" An Aerosmith lyric), It should be noted that currently in 2013 that birth control drugs are so thoroughly in water supplies in urban areas including university campus water that one does not have to ingest birth control directly as a drug to be influenced adversely...
  All Cancers, Note please: calcium is the element that is fabricated into progesterone to make birth control drugs-at those doses it causes Cancer...It is teratogenic which is how children get born with cancer(which means the cancer is CONGENITAL NOT GENETIC)...Also causes

children to be born gender dysphoric or adrenal gland failure(aids)...There are herbal(lower dose) forms of calcium which cause celibate behaviours but do not cause cancer...ie: Vitus Agnus Castus (an herb)...

I repeat, Cancer is caused by birth control drugs...Hence why it is so common today...It also transfers between couples...The woman will excrete the drug onto the man... Prostate Cancer...

http://en.wikipedia.org/wiki/Birth_control_pill Some of this wikipedia on the birth control pill is dubious...However, it should be noted that Japan blocked the sale of the pill for almost 40 years, which is why rates of cancer & Aids(both are adrenal gland blocks or failures due to blocks), why the rates of these syndromes are so low in Japan!

The pill(a Calcium mega dose), came onto many markets between 1955 & 1961...Which is why so many people started to get sick between those times especially...The whole poliovirus causing Cancer or aids thing is just a cover story for the fact that the birth control pill was causing aids & cancer & gender dysphorias...

Why a cover story? Because men in particular, & most doctors were men back then, would prefer to take the risk of giving their wife breast cancer or ovarian cancer or other cancers, than have a plethora of children they have to work their whole life to pay for...

Note:If women would stop insisting of having a plethora of children, especially ones they cannot pay for themselves, then men might stop making them take birth control drugs...This is my opinion as a woman, who doesn't have any children, & who has a very happy life & happy husband...

*Not to mention the fact that the law says, even if a man divorces a woman, he still has to pay for her & the children she insisted on having, even though he has moved on due to unhappiness...

**This is all my opinion, & may peeve some people...That is understood...

More on Calcium Excess: Overbreeding of the Mother leading to Gender Dysphoria in the Offspring...

*So we know that Spleen damage can cause a Phosphorus excess(A PLUS element excess)...So logically, we could theorize that Adrenal Gland damage might cause a calcium excess in the Adrenal Gland...We know birth control drugs are Calcium...We know Calcium excess causes gender dysphoria, Cancer & Aids(adrenal gland failure)...Now...If a woman is Overbred...Way too many children...We know that the later offspring can have gender dysphoria...Calcium excess...This can be caused by 2 factors...1)Adrenal gland damage leading to Calcium excess in the Mother being passed on teratogenically(during pregnancy) to the fetus/baby...2)Or, the mother got tired of having so many children so she started taking birth control pills patches or injections, causing the Calcium excess, but then got pregnant anyway-then the Calcium excess gets passed on as well...

United States On June 10, 1957, Australia Jan. 1961, Germany June 1961, Britain dec. 4, 1961, France dec. 28, 1967, Japan June 1999

Do you know what those dates are? Above? Those are the dates that the birth control pill got approved in each of those countries...(source wikipedia on birth control drugs)...

Notice anything? The US approved it first...Japan approved it last...Which country has tons of cancer? The US...Which country has very little cancer...Japan...
Enough said...

Grove Body Part Chart

Organ	Minus Element	Plus Element
Thyroid	Zinc	Lead
Thymus	Manganese	Iron
Lungs & Lymph Nodes	Titanium	Aluminum
Heart	Potassium	Aurum
Kidneys	Carbon	Nitrogen
Pancreas	Selenium	Sulphur
Liver	Oxygen	Hydrogen
Spleen	Copper	Phosphorus
Adrenal Gland	Iodine	Calcium
Gallbladder	Magnesium	Mercury
Colon	Fluorine	Bismuth

Mental:Calcium excess can also cause a mental blocking-your body feels one thing but your brain is thinking a different thought...There is a disconnect between brain thought & body feeling...or a time delay...This can cause inappropriate reactions, where you are reacting to something from earlier in the day, later on, say at work, where it is completely inappropriate... (you have inappropriate sexual impulses in the workplace, that are really a time delayed reaction to something perfectly normal at home, earlier in the day, or the night before...)(note

Nettle herb steeped into a tea(or boiled), is an easy to source, great way to get Iodine, which cleans out Calcium excess & can help to correct those inappropriate time delayed moments)...

Elements:where to find,

Adrenal Gland: Iodine (a Minus Element): Vinpocetine, Vincristine, Chemotherapy drugs, Madagascar Periwinkle (*tea),
*HearAll hearing capsules also *VeinGuard capsules(Both from NaturalCare in Oregon), Seaweed salad, Kelp supplements, Fish, Odewalla green smoothy drinks contain Dulse (30%), Arame is a sea vegetable that contains Tons of iodine-see my Arame recipe on my Medical Arts blog at http://www.grovecanada.com
Red Wine contains Iodine(they call that resveratrol in red grapes but it is an iodine element), the drug Warfarin is an Iodine drug, as is the rat poison also called Warfarin...
Iodine is also found in the annual nettle or stinging nettle plant...(used in herbals)...
Raspberry LEAF can be drunk as a tea & is an IODINE element...(the fruit itself is more of an Oxygen element-see Liver)...
More iodine things: Nettle Leaf steeped in a french press(ours is Bodum), makes a great IODINE tea...It really seems to clear out breast lumps in particular, & is easier to find than Madagscar Periwinkle, another herb than can be made into a tea, which cleans out Cancer/calcium excesses in a stronger way...(be forewarned-iodine teas & things will make you sleepy initially, then afterwards you feel energetic...But prepare for the sleepiness by taking the day off work if you drink some...) A bloody nose or bleediness means to cut back or stop for a while...Taking rest breaks while taking stuff ensures you don't overdose...(like 2 weeks)...
Warfarin also known commercially as Coumadin is a drug that is an Iodine drug...It is also a rat poison...Warfarin can cause photosensitivity, as well as DEMENTIA...Warfarin is commonly prescribed & then the patient is forgotten...There are people in retirement homes or old age homes still taking warfarin despite the fact that they have developed dementia...People with dementia should not be taking warfarin anymore...People are told that warfarin is for their heart, but in reality Iodine based drugs are anti-cancer, & those clots they mention or warn about, would be Calcium deposits which are Cancer deposits in technical terms...So all the troubles associated with chemo can also go along with Warfarin...It is a very dangerous drug & should be stopped in the long term...The family of the person taking warfarin will have to step in as current protocols leave people on warfarin far after it has wreaked havoc, with diarrhea & dementia being the first signs it has been overused...

Adrenal Gland: Calcium (a Plus Element): Progesterone based Birth Control drugs patches or injections like *Depo Provera, Milk, Vitus Agnus castus, Saltpeter, Depo Provera

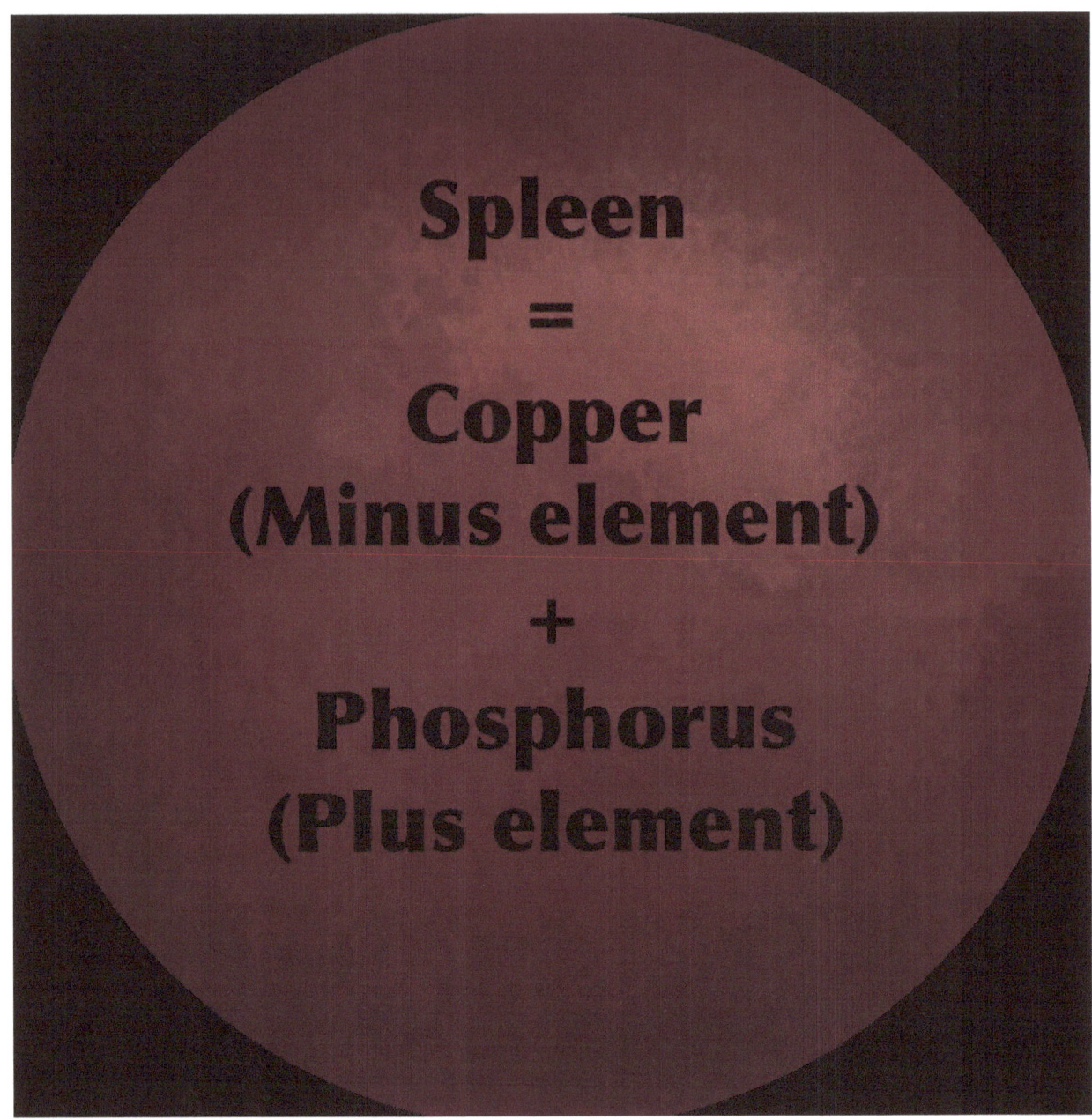

Spleen=Copper(Minus element)+Phosphorus(Plus element)

http://www.grovecanada.com/blog/2013/10/work-connecting-the-nose-the-spleen-the-globus-pallidusmapping-the-brain-ideas.html

Spleen to Globus Palladus to Nose Minus Copper with Plus Phosphorus

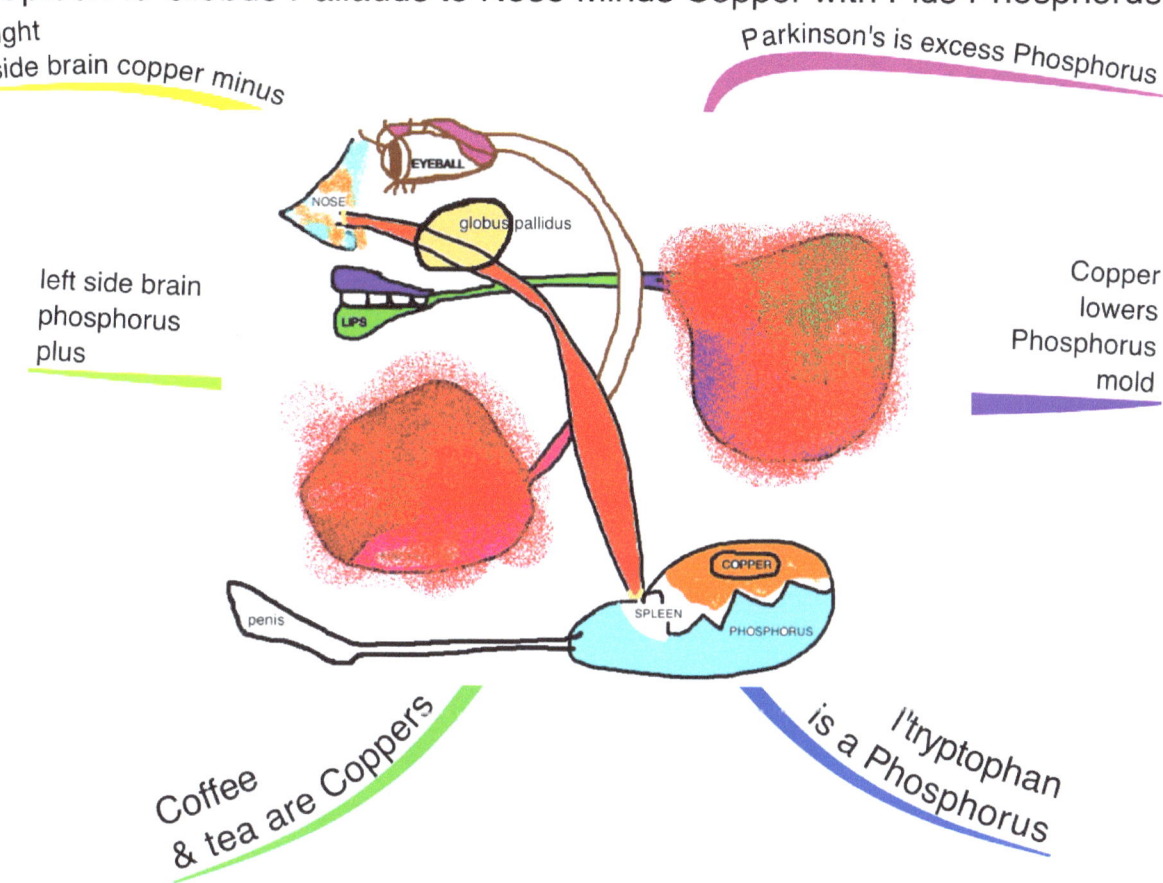

right side brain copper minus

Parkinson's is excess Phosphorus

left side brain phosphorus plus

Copper lowers Phosphorus mold

Coffee & tea are Coppers

l'tryptophan is a Phosphorus

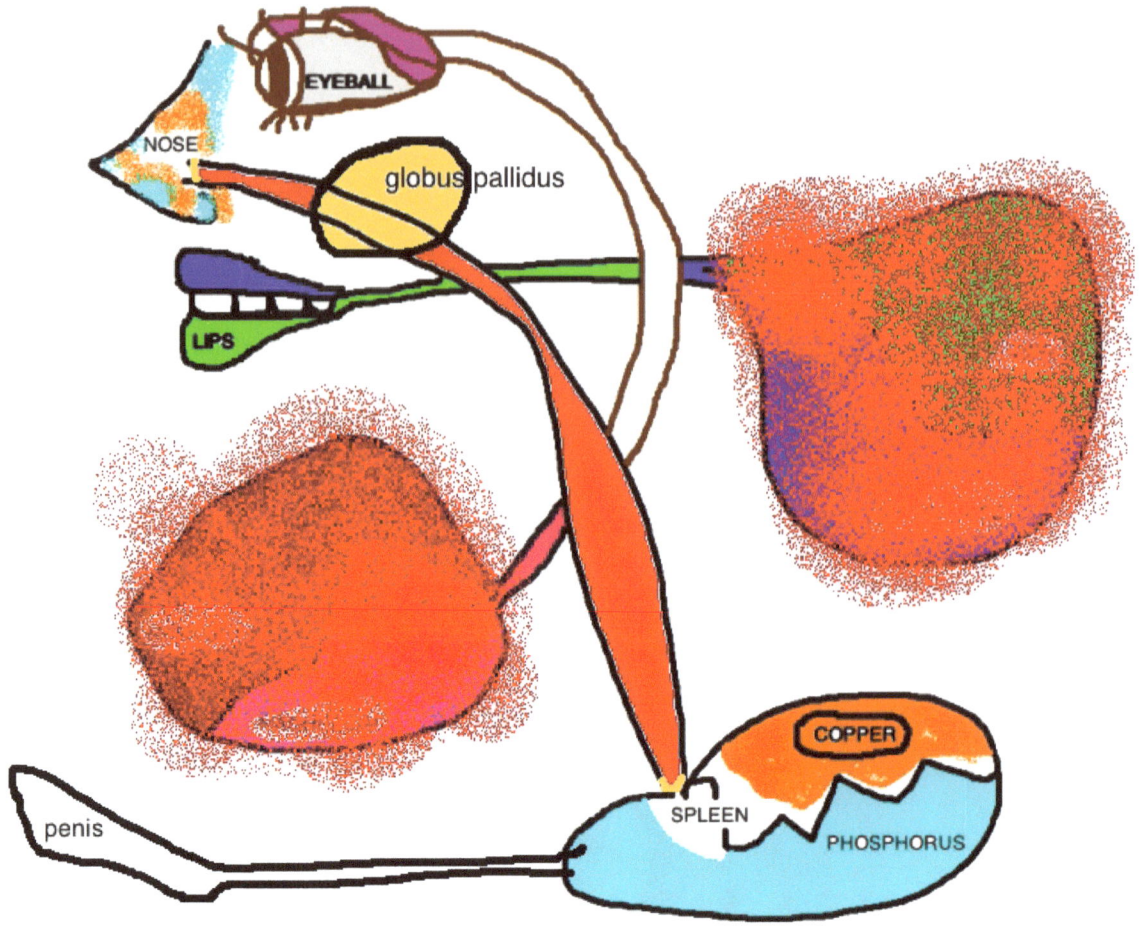

Spleen:

Too much Copper (a Minus Element): Incredible amounts of energy sexuality doping at Olympics, rash decisions made while speeding through time, can't slow down, accidents, hyperactive acid reflux is also excess copper(think black coffee on an empty stomach)

Spleen:

 Too much Phosphorus (a Plus Element): Parkinson's disease, Salmonella... Also tremor is caused by too much Phosphorus...A side effect of too much Hydrogen (like alcohol) is it will or may increase Phosphorus as well in the Spleen causing a tremor...Hand Tremor...Muscle Tremors...Slow, placid, unfeeling moods...

1   Hot Straws & how I came up with my understanding of Parkinson's ... Jul 24, 2013 ... People ask me how I got into medical research...How did I come up with my ideas ? It is kind of a long story, but today I mentioned one of my ...
http://www.grovecanada.com/blog/2013/07/hot-straws-how-i-came-up-with-my-understanding-of-parkinsons-disease.html

2   Grove Body Part Chart, a video introduction by Sari Grove, & some ... Jun 23, 2013 ...
Some proofs that go with my Grove Body Part Chart: Spleen, Copper as remedy &
Parkinson's disease(caused by Phosphorus excess):.
http://www.grovecanada.com/blog/2013/06/grove-body-part-chart-a-video-
introduction-by-sari-grove-some-outside-support-for-some-of-my-theorie.html

3   The Iatrogenic Effect: otherwise known as medicine making you sick ... Sep 4, 2012 ...
Parkinson's disease may develop...An injured spleen needs copper...I recommend
chelated copper supplements for Parkinson's disease, ...
http://www.grovecanada.com/blog/2012/09/tuberculosis-cement-or-concrete-dust-
from-construction-sites-buildings-contains-aluminum-other-elemental-particles-which-
c.html

This is where the Minus Plus designation of the elements come in...If you have a PLUS element
excess in one organ, there are chances that you will also have a PLUS element excess
in organs nearby...

Once again, Salmonella(food poisoning) is a Phosphorus excess...(treat with Copper things like
coffee-hand grind your coffee beans & the oils are so much stronger right away)...

Mold is Phosphorus...

It's opposite is Copper...

It affects the SPLEEN organ...

Copper is found easily in really good coffee...(Jamaican Blue Mountain coffee is good-expensive
but good for copper)

You can eat a coffee bean straight...Like just chew it...

You can just hammer coffee beans to grind them...

Manual coffee bean grinders are fun(& not noisy & cheap) 'cause you get lots of arm exercise
then you really appreciate the tiny powder you made plus you won't drink too much coffee
'cause you can't...(too tired)...

You can also order Colloidal copper as a liquid on Amazon...It is clear & tasteless & you can put
it in anything you usually drink even hot drinks...

You can wear copper against your skin...Make sure it is fresh copper because it loses its power
fast...Change the jewelry when you sense you have absorbed all the copper in it...Put on a new
one, necklace, bracelet...

You can put coffee grains instant or grinds into your bathtub...Use alot alot alot...The better the coffee the more copper...(cheap coffee can have lower copper but higher magnesium...)

All this copper will clean the mold out of your body...

You can leave copper stuff lying around in your home to get rid of airborne & other mold...

Be VERY careful when cleaning mold...Very careful...Wear a mask & gloves & take breaks & strip clothing off after cleaning & take plenty of hot showers & scrub scrub scrub...

Get some scrub gloves, exfoliating gloves for the bath & scrub with those...

Fresh air, Oxygen & exercise will help...

Elements:where to find,

Spleen,

Phosphorus (a Plus Element):Old cheese, (Lapis Lazuli the blue stone contains phosphorus), Blue Mold(an injured spleen will be Phosphorus heavy-like in Parkinson's disease or tremor conditions)...Phosphorus is also found in L'Tryptophan which is a supplement or found in heated milk or in a Thanksgiving dinner...It is very settling & can help one to sleep...Feed someone who is sleep described an impromptu Thanksgiving meal, any time of the year-also has applications for epileptics-see the Colon Page for those ideas...tryptophan means phosphorus...
**Serotonin is a Phosphorus element...Valerian Root is a Phosphorus element...

Copper (a Minus Element):Coffee, Colloidal Copper Clear Liquid Supplement, Somali 'chatt' (phonetic)-cat grass-contains copper, Tea, Black tea, Green tea (Note: http://
www.Hotstraw.com
invented a straw you can put in coffee or tea so your teeth don't turn yellow from drinking too much-it also works for tremor Parkinson patients who tremor too much to
hold their hot drink steady to drink it-these are important because people with Parkinson's or resting muscle tremors need copper & also they don't want yellow teeth from drinking coffee all the time!)...Also Copper is called Tyrosine in bodybuilding supplements...Dopamine is copper
http://muhc.ca/newsroom/news/caffeine-may-ease-parkinsons-symptoms
*Rose petals used in herbals as a tea is a Copper element...
**Ritalin is a COPPER element based drug like cocaine, crystal meth & coffee or tea...You could theoretically use Ritalin to treat Parkinson's disease or tremor, since Parkinson's & other tremors are Phosphorus overload which is opposite to Copper in the SPLEEN...
Neat trick:Take a bath in coffee grains if you have Parkinson's, a tremor, or any Phosphorus overload in the Spleen...(a blow to the spleen can cause a Phosphorus overload too)...
 I used Tim Horton's coarse ground coffee in a tin...It's cheap $6.99 a can & so you don't care about using alot...Coffee makes a good scrub too-body & face! (you lose weight too when you bathe in it)...Coffee baths give you a tanned healthy look too!

**Serotonin INHIBITORS are Copper elements (since Phosphorus is serotonin & an inhibitor means the opposite to...)*Most ANTI-depressants are based on Copper(which is opposite to Phosphorus in the Spleen)...

*Anti-depressants, which are basically Copper elements, can cause all sorts of side-effects including bipolar-like episodes...

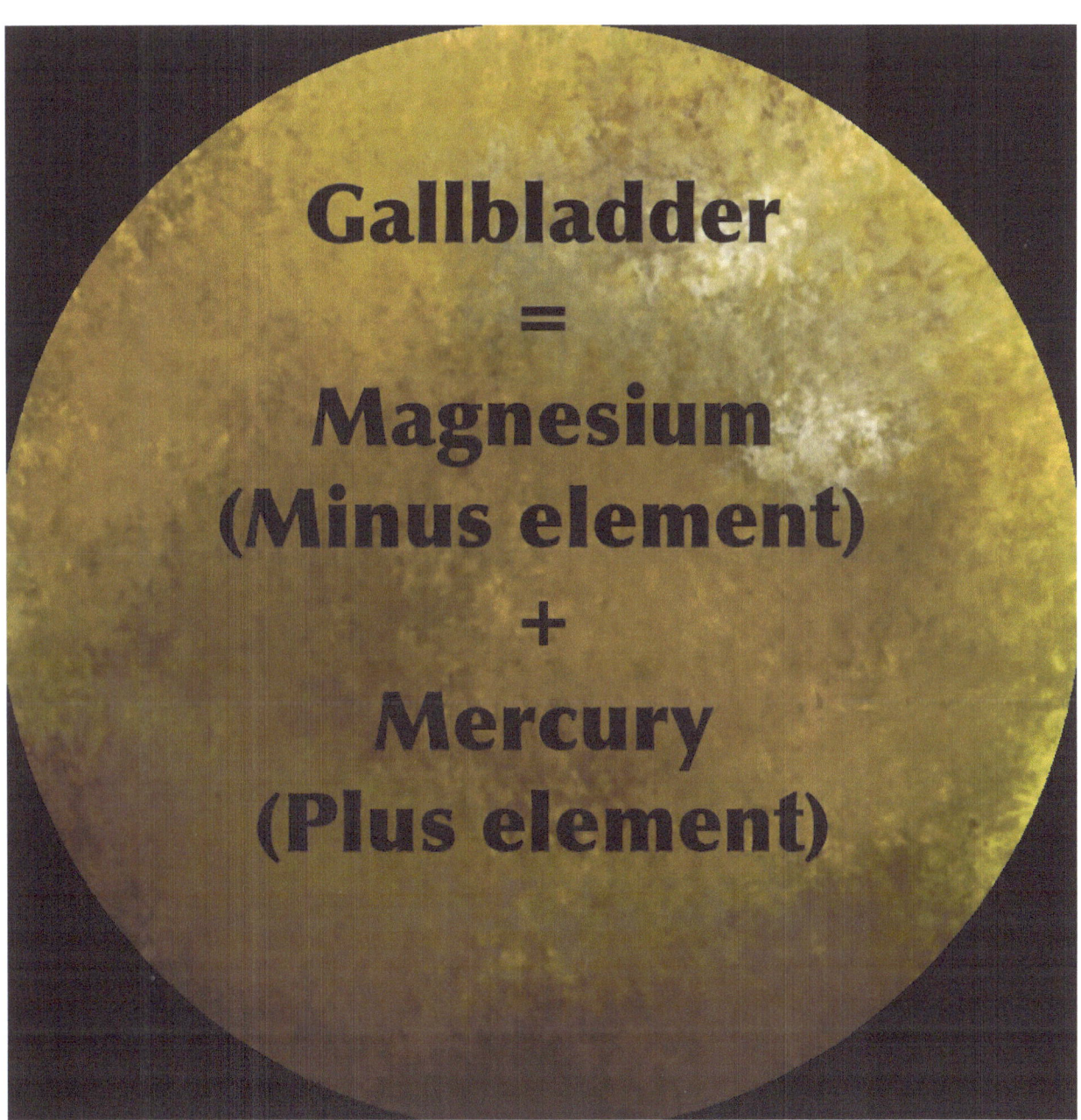

Gallbladder=Magnesium(Minus element)+Mercury (Plus element)

Broca's Area speech to lips to Gallbladder to Mercury plus Magnesium Minus

Cartilage & Joints
are built up with Mercury Plus

Arthritis & Polio
are Magnesium excess

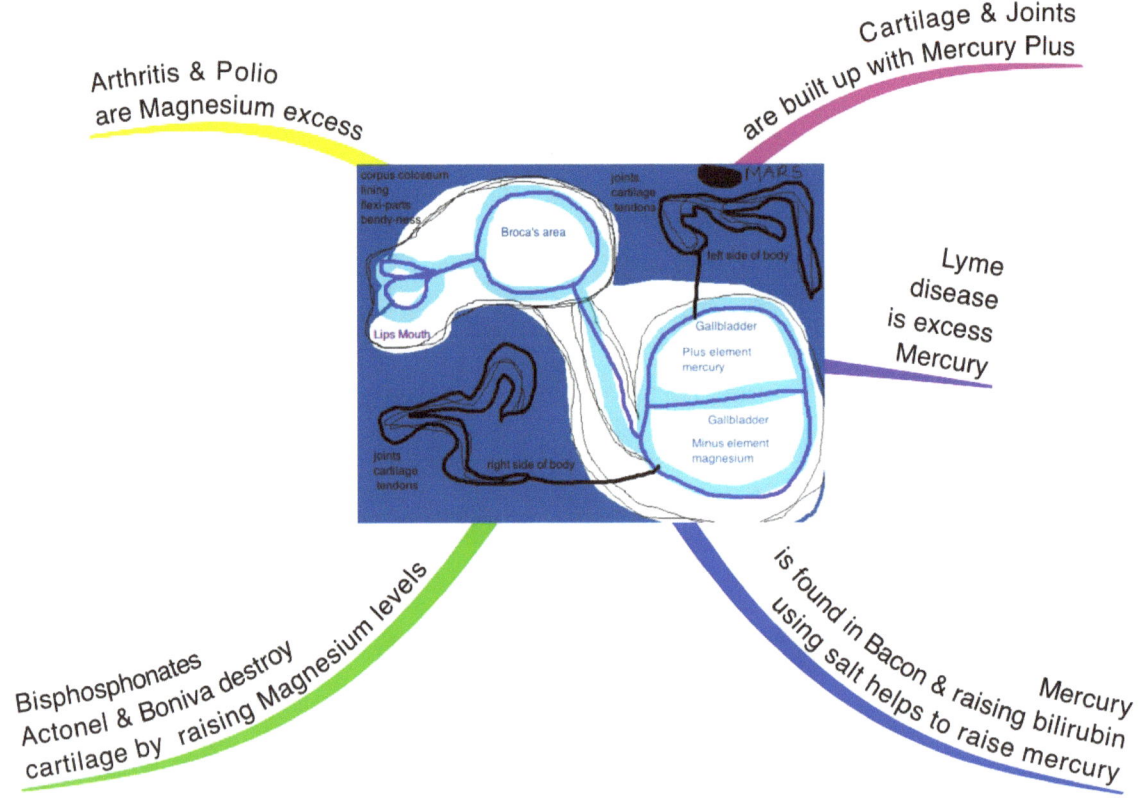

Lyme
disease
is excess
Mercury

Bisphosphonates
Actonel & Boniva destroy
cartilage by raising Magnesium levels

Mercury
is found in Bacon & raising bilirubin
using salt helps to raise mercury

http://www.grovecanada.com/blog/2013/10/brocas-area-the-speaking-mouth-the-gallbladder.html

Broca's area in the brain controls speech, attaches to the lips & mouth, & also connects to the Gallbladder with its mercury magnesium opposing twins...

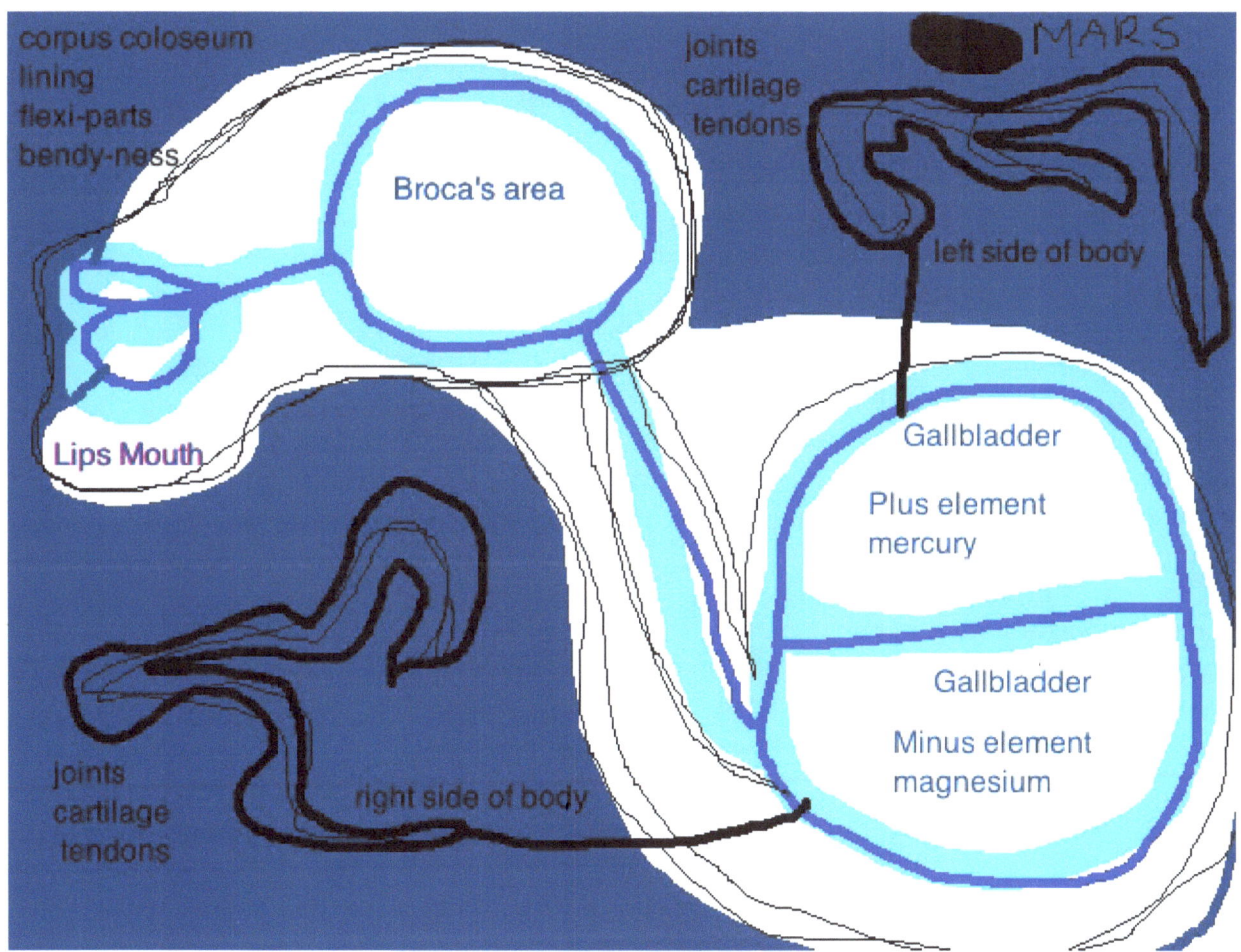

Gallbladder:

 Too much Magnesium (a Minus Element) =Stills disease -congenital, Arthritis, Rheumatoid, Stiffness in Joints, Chondromalacia of the Patella, Lack of cartilage, Low Bilirubin, Jaw pain,
 *Need for
hip jaw elbow shoulder knee ankle replacement(drugs like Boniva & Actonel & other bisphosphonate drugs CAUSE excess magnesium thus degrading cartilage & also causing

fractures & causing need for joint replacement surgeries-Class Action lawsuits are being served as we speak)), Chondromalacia of the Patella (knees that click when you bend), Necrosis of the jaw(jaw death), Aches & Pains, back pain, Bell's Palsy(facial tendons are degraded in Bell's), fibromylagia...Osteoarthritis...Encephalomyelitis(degradation of brain tendons let's say in the Broca's area of the brain where speech is handled & lips & mouth function)...
IBS irritable bowel syndrome is usually too much poohing or diarrhea related to magnesium excess 'cause magnesium is a strong laxative!

I'd like to note here:That Obesity is NOT arthritis...What I mean to say is that a mechanical pressure on your joints due to overweightness is not the same as an imbalance in your Gallbladder typified by a Magnesium excess that causes degradation of cartilage...You can create arthritis by taking too many magnesium supplements, it destroys your cartilage & it is very painful...Some people are born with this imbalance or exercise or work too much & create this imbalance...Being very heavy weightwise can cause pain as well, but this is not really rheumatoid arthritis...This is being overweight & can be fixed by losing weight...Not all pain in your joints is a magnesium imbalance...Whilst someone with a true arthritis needs to add mercury to their diet by raising their bilirubin levels & eating foods that do this, someone who is overweight & has pain in their knees should NOT do that...They simply need to lose weight & that will remove the cause of the pain...Which is why heavy people who know they are too heavy should not declare they have arthritis, nor should they be treated as such nor be given drugs to treat that...They just need to focus on why they are overweight, the physical & psychological reasons behind that, & deal with the issue of weight....In women, much obesity today is due to Calcium excess due to birth control drugs...(in men, Calcium excess actually causes loss of weight, so that is not true for men)...In men, it might be the Nitrogen excess caused by heavy drinking that bulks up the weight...But in either case, the extra weight has nothing to do with a Magnesium excess which is what a true arthritis is-unless they are self-medicating, & then you are looking at a rebound ailment...(a rebound ailment might be one that is caused by someone overcorrecting another problem)...

**Broca's area of the brain controls the mouth & attaches to the Gallbladder...So when you have too much Magnesium & not enough mercury, all those body parts get involved...In more severe cases, TASTE can get lost...Loss of sensation of taste...Related to lack of Mercury, excess Magnesium...(solution is to RAISE mercury bilirubin by eating salty things, peameal canadian bacon, fast food, Kentucky Fried Chicken-YUP, just say I said it was ok!)!

1   Update on fixing Cartilage Degeneration, Rheumatoid Arthritis, Back ... Nov 22, 2012 ... I spoke at length to Marie-Claude Brutus Lopez in Ottawa at Health Canada...I reported a full length history as best as I could about Actonel ...
http://www.grovecanada.com/blog/2012/11/update-on-fixing-cartilage-degeneration-rheumatoid-arthritis-back-pains-due-to-slipped-discs-that-so.html

2   Creutzfeldt-Jakob disease, Mad Cow disease, Gallstones, Jaundice ... Feb 6, 2013 ... Too much mercury & you can get gallstones... Too much magnesium & you can get rheumatoid arthritis... The gallbladder is in charge of making ...
http://www.grovecanada.com/blog/2013/02/creutzfeldt-jakob-disease-mad-cow-disease-gallstones-jaundice-stuttering-eye-twitches-adhd-autism.html

3   Download 118071034-Grove-Body-Part-Chart - The Grove Body ... rheumatoid arthritis needs more mercury, they need to raise bilirubin ...

4   http://www.grovecanada.com/files/118071034-grove-body-part-chart.pdf

1   http://www.upright-health.com/syringomyelia.html Syringomyelia can be a result of Meningitis, Meningitis is a lesser form of POLIO... I now think these are all Fluorine excess syndromes, due to the paralytic nature of the symptoms-paralysis as a symptom goes with Fluorine excess)...

Gallbladder:

Too much Mercury (a Plus Element): High Bilirubin, Constipation, Communication difficulty, Mute-ness, Autism, ADHD, ADD, Violence... Violent behaviour including bullying...Violent, violence...(being very physical-which does not include aggression-aggression is high Nitrogen which is different)...But high mercury also means strong cartilage development...Good joints! Stuttering is also a sign of high Mercury levels...Swine flu(H1N1 is the new word for that) is also mercury excess...(so treat with magnesium things-lavender tea is a magnesium thing btw)... Asperger's is like autism & ADHD, an mercury excess too...

Author's Note on Friday January 3, 2014:(Sari Grove) Ok, this whole next piece is under dispute...In my own head...Now that I reread what I have written, I once again am having doubts about my own work...The source of my confusion is that my mother-in-law told me that when she got Meningitis as a child in Winnipeg(many children died of Polio back then, there-50 maybe, in 1948-1949), they gave her some antibiotics, she was sick for 2 weeks, then got better...The fact that they gave her antibiotics(a Selenium drug for the Pancreas that lowers blood sugar levels there) indicates to me that Meningitis(& Polio by proxy) responded to a Minus element drug...But I have said further that I think meningitis & polio are Minus element excess...
But a Minus excess would not respond to a Minus element drug...So I think I am confused...

My mother-in-law's later life presents as a Fluorine excess syndrome...Later paralysis, a Fluorine excess, mimicking ALS...But is that what I see a RESULT of the treatment for Meningitis, NOT the disease itself???

Is the syringomyelia, leading to arachnoiditis, is that really the RESULT of heavy antibiotic treatment? Is that the POST-meningitis syndrome, not the syndrome itself?

A POST syndrome would be a syndrome that results from the TREATMENT, not from the disease...

Gets treated with a barrage of antibiotics & the patient is left bereft with weakened tendons? With weakened spinal cord connections that can lead to ruptures???(I'm putting this aside for a moment, will get back to it)...

New: Lyme Encephalopathy(encephalopathy just means brain involvement, in this case with Lyme, a Mercury excess in Broca's area which controls speech & lips & mouth, & Gallbladder, so people with Mercury excess will have gunk, mercury, gunking up their speech-like dyslexic conversations...Also jaundice, maybe a yellow look to their face skin...)

(treatments for Lyme that involve Magnesium, the opposite to Mercury in the gallbladder have been very successful...)http://www.wellsphere.com/lyme-disease-article/evidence-magnesium-deficiency-is-related-to-lyme-disease/981959

The Lyme disease tick is very attracted to people with high Mercury levels, which is why, by lowering Mercury levels, by Raising Magnesium levels, you can get rid of them...It...

Lyme disease is 7 times more common among Asians, which points to a Mercury excess common & particular to Asian peoples...(*Mercury levels can be elevated due to eating significant amounts of pork-which is a common food preference to the Asian race)...http://www.jle.com/en/revues/bio_rech/mrh/e-docs/00/03/FD/D1/article.phtml(original study showing efficacy of magnesium treatment for Lyme...Note:lowering sugar/sulphur levels in the Pancreas is traditional therapy called antibiotics-antibiotics are just Selenium/garlic...By lowering sugar/sulphur levels, that progresses down to the Gallbladder & lowers mercury levels too...So that helps too...)

-I'd add to this note about Lyme disease, that Asian people also have a much greater tendency towards diabetes, which is a Sugar/Sulphur excess in the Pancreas...The combination of Sugar/Sulphur excess tendency plus Mercury excess tendency, due to a preference for sugar & pork eating culturally, would make Asian people very attractive to a hungry tick...Which is why by lowering sugar levels with antibiotics(selenium or garlic), & lowering mercury levels with Magnesium things(oral epsom salts work), you can kill the ticks...

-However, AFTER you have gotten rid of all the ticks, you may be left with an arthritis like condition which is actually a MAGNESIUM EXCESS...So with Lyme disease, you have to decide, are you at the stage where you need to kill the initial tick infection, or are you at the AFTER phase where you need to repair your cartilage???(*Hint:If you are in the After phase, then you actually need to ADD Mercury things to your diet-like bacon or raise your bilirubin with salt to ease the pain...)

Treatment for Lyme disease is the OPPOSITE to treatment for the after effects of Lyme disease...Know that big big difference!

Heavy doses of magnesium plus antibiotics surely cause arthritis, paralysis, fibromyalgia-are we seeing a drug induced effect in this "chronic Lyme disease" syndrome thing?

 *http://www.lymebook.com/top10book This book talks about the 10 best practices for curing Lyme disease...

Lyme disease is for sure Mercury excess...However...If you OVERTREAT Lyme disease, you will get The whole arthritic thing...This is where Iatrogenic effect comes in...IATROGENIC means something caused by physician intervention...This "Chronic" Lyme disease problem seems to be an Iatrogenic effect, possibly caused by OVERmedicating Lyme...

 Ok...We know Lyme disease is a Mercury excess...Raised bilirubin(mercury Hg) in the Gallbladder...
 So...It gets treated usually with antibiotics which are Selenium Se(which lowers blood sugar levels in the Pancreas)...
 Excessive antibiotics, or even just a regular dose of antibiotics(think tons of raw garlic in your body), can cause diarrhea, or violent diarrhea, depending on the overdose or size of the body...*Many women get overdosed because a male doctor will estimate for a man's size-this is not a mistake exactly, just a natural tendency that could be solved by more women entering medical school...
 Ok so now we have diarrhea induced by antibiotics, given to cure Lyme...
 DIARRHEA can cause arthritis like symptoms, cartilage joint problem pain symptoms...Yup diarrhea...(You can induce diarrhea just by taking too much magnesium too)...

 I think this "Chronic Lyme disease thing" is caused by the antibiotics used to treat the real Lyme...An iatrogenic effect...
  ****Note:That type of problem, the joint pain thing needs to be treated with Mercury things like bacon, or Rudraksha beads, or adding Salt to the diet daily, or eat junk & fast food that is salty-anything that RAISES bilirubin, hotdogs, spam...

:http://www.medscape.com/viewarticle/763458 Just to clarify...if you have UNTREATED Lyme disease then you have a MERCURY excess in the GALLBLADDER & you will be exhibiting symptoms similar to ADHD attention deficit hyperactivity disorder

(ed. note:Um...More precisely, you have a Mercury excess, then ticks are attracted to you more because of that delicious mercury excess-you smell like bacon for example which raises mercury levels in the gallbladder-then the tick bites you & starts feeding off your mercury, mmm delicious, then as it saps your mercury you start feeling tired...However, to kill the tick you have to take magnesium plus antibiotics plus any other Minus element from my Chart, 'cause Minus elements all line up as cleansing things in the body parts...This is a truer picture of symptoms...Bugs are hard to pin down!)

*So either you have Lyme disease, a Mercury excess, or you could have treatment symptoms, which are the OPPOSITE(a magnesium excess) to Lyme...Know the difference!

(ADHD symptoms are like, you're typing & you keep making dyslexic mistakes, your verbal sentences come out wrong, in the wrong order, you feel violent or are violent, jaundice...Magnesium excess symptoms are arthritis pain joint pain sore jaw back pain poohing too much...These are opposite things...)

More about Lyme:Lyme is usually treated with antibiotics(lowers blood sugar in the Pancreas like garlic does-antibiotics are an Selenium element)...But Lyme can persist even after treatment...This is why I think that Lyme is a Mercury excess in the Gallbladder...On my chart, adding a Minus element in one body part will also trigger other Minus elements in other body parts...So Selenium antibiotics will trigger Magnesium too...Which is why antibiotics work for so many things...But you do need to get specific...To really cure the common cold, you need an Oxygen thing...To really cure Lyme you need a Magnesium thing...

You may notice Lyme resembles Swine flu H1N1, which is also a Mercury excess...You may notice Lyme resembles autism ADHD which is also a mercury excess...

So add a magnesium thing to your life to eradicate all of Lyme...See below for where to find magnesium elements...

Ok back to POLIO: I am revisiting my views on Polio...Polio has paralysis as a symptom, which then says it is a Fluorine excess not even in the Gallbladder! Phew! Paralysis type things are Fluorine excesses in the Colon(according to how I am simplifying things into my Grove Body Part Chart)...Polio also has throat problems, esophageal problems, which are iconically characteristic as well of fluorine excess in the Colon...That means meninigitis as well is a Fluorine excess, like ALS (Lou Gehrig's)...

Citations: www.medicalnewstoday.com/articles/155580
Polio, or poliomyelitis, is a highly contagious viral infection that can lead to paralysis, (which also speaks to Typhus & Cholera which are also fluorine excess)...
http://www.nofluoride.com/what_doctors_donot_tell.cfmPolio resembles fluoride poisoning (Anterior horn cell damage in both)
This link above speaks to the fact that fluoride poisoning causes anterior horn cell damage...It also states that Polio ALSO causes Anterior horn cell damage...This helps my case in saying that Polio is a fluorine excess...(also that fluorine causes paralysis in high doses)...
"which explains why polio victims are paralyzed or suffer from impaired motor function"(from article above)...
Also,
"Gastrointestinal disturbances, often referred to as IBS...as they are in the Chronic Fluoride Toxicity Syndrome." (diarrhea type problems are another sign of fluorine excess, though you need other signs to confirm since diarrhea can be other things too-though this is increasing confirmation that Polio, Typhus & Cholera are all Fluorine excess in the Colon)
BACKGROUND TO FLUORIDATION. ... "On Dec 28, 1956 the City of Winnipeg began to add fluoride to the city's water supply system for a future of healthier teeth." Now this is where my head turns a bit...

Discussion:If children in Winnipeg contracted Polio & meningitis(meningitis is now sometimes referred to as a feature of Polio as opposed to a separate thing), in 1948 & 1949, then that was Before the water there was fluoridated...So we could say that the cause of this fluorine excess disease is NOT artificial fluoridation...

Then how? Well, regular water, untreated can carry high amounts of natural fluorine...They see it in Florida all the time, they call it Red Tide, & many species of sea creatures die & wash up on shore(hence the red tide designation)-this is often when the water is warmer as fluorine becomes stronger in heat...
  Now we could posit that the natural water in Winnipeg became naturally overfluoridated in 1948-49...
(was it hotter that summer?Have to check)...

ok so July 1948 (Winnipeg) temperature high was 25.7
August 1948 (high)26.4
Sept 1948 (high) 24.0

let's look at other years in Winnipeg to compare:

!n 1947 the high in Sept was only 17.9
In 1949 Sept was only 18.3
1950 Sept was 19.08
In 1946 Sept was 18.3(the high temperature)
http://climate.weather.gc.ca/climateData/monthlydata_e.html?timeframe=3&Prov=MAN&StationID=3698&mlyRange=1938-01-01%7C2007-11-01&Year=1948&Month=01&Day=01 (These historical temperatures are courtesy of the link above-Gov't of Canada Climate weather data download) These numbers were all in Celsius by the way...(for Winnipeg Richardson Airport, latitude 49.92, longitude -97.23, elevation 238.70, Climate identifier 5023222)

Randomly looking at other Septembers in Winnipeg history,
 1940 has a 24.0 high, like the one in 1948 when the children got Polio...
But not until 1948 does the September temperature get up back to that 1940 high temperature...

24.1 Celsius=75.380 Fahrenheit (the Sept high for 1948 Winnipeg)...
http://www.metric-conversions.org/temperature/celsius-to-fahrenheit.htm

*the year before, 1947, Sept., was 17.9 (high for Sept.) which is 64.220 Fahrenheit...

A difference of 11.6 degrees Fahrenheit...warmer...

The year 1948 distinguished itself from the 8 years previous of colder Septembers (1940 had a similar high), until again in 1952 the high in Sept. was 21.1 C(69.98 F)...
Interestingly there was another outbreak of Polio in 1952-53 in Winnipeg...

www.glenbow.org/50s/fear_eng.htm

"The most feared was polio. ... Through 1952 and 1953 the western provinces had a major epidemic, severest in Winnipeg but Calgary also had several hundred cases."

Could a 10 or 11 degree rise in temperature in the month of September in Winnipeg cause Natural Fluorine levels to rise in the water supply there???

Could this have triggered the Polio outbreaks there?

(remember that charcoal filtering which offsets fluorine in water were probably not as sophisticated as they are now...)

Well...Let's see...
environment.about.com/od/redtidesfaq/f/red_tide_causes.htm
"Scientists have correlated the increase of Pacific red tides and other harmful algae blooms with a rise in ocean temperature of approximately one degree..."
Ok, so ONE DEGREE can cause the harmful Red Tide that kills sealife so easily!!!

So yes, we can say that a rise in temperature by a 11.6 degrees from one September in Winnipeg 1947, to the next September 1948, could cause harmful Red Tide-LIKE effects in the water supply, which are characterized by a rise in (natural) FLUORINE levels which became deadly at those higher temperatures, & were not offset well enough by water charcoal filtering...(which neutralizes if sufficient, fluorine which is acidic)...

So we have some clues about how Polio(& Typhus & Cholera & ALS & Crohn's disease & Fabry (an orphan illness with progressive hearing loss & IBS) & hearing loss & IBS(poohing too much) & severe dehydration, as well as insomnia, excess domesticity(no independent spirit), & other slow progressive paralytic disorders...

www.winnipegfreepress.com/local/fast-and-furious-polio...
"THE polio outbreak in 1948-'49 on the western shore of Hudson Bay spread fast and furious among a people... -" Local - Winnipeg Free Press.

Ideas about this discovery? I guess, charcoal filters are a good thing...Be careful what water you drink or swim in...Hotter Septembers are not always a good thing...Artificial fluoridation is not always the cause of fluoride excess diseases...
  **(one might assume that artificial fluoridation is what happens AFTER charcoal filtering which filters out many things bad & good, & so they put some fluorine back in at the end of the process, after they have removed the natural fluorines)...

Also, that despite the fact that antibiotics may have been given for meningitis (or polio which is related closely), that That was not why some children got better...That was a red herring so to speak, a false clue...

  More correctly, seeing that Polio/Meningitis is probably a Fluorine excess, then the antidote or balancing act would be a Bismuth, Indium (Wild Indigo Root is an easy to get Indium Bismuth type thing) or even just plain activated charcoal powder...(indium is like Charcoal just stronger, but a different name & box on the Periodic Table of Elements)...

Comment:Which is why Global Warming may seem like fun to cold Canadians, but in fact every degree of warmer weather can cause Epilepsy, ALS, Polio, Typhus, Cholera, Hearing loss, Crohn's disease, IBS, Insomnia, Double Aortic Arch(Distended heart), & other FLUORINE Excess related diseases, which are usually seen in colder climates...Which answer an earlier question of mine which was:"why are so many children in Ottawa Ontario showing epilepsy & seizure disorders which used to be rare in Canada?"

Answer, because global warming is warming our waters & causing fluorine excess problems because fluorine becomes deadly in too warm waters...

*****(Some ideas concerning predispositions based on location geographically-an ongoing study (Note: I have noticed 2 dispositions particular to the Australian...
1) Mercury excess-which can lead to violent tendency & a fictional outlook on real issues(but great cartilage development & physicality)
2) 2)Fluorine excess-which can lead to loudness spoken words, which is really a slight hearing loss(fluorine also keeps you awake at night, causes diarrhea, epilepsy, & ALS)...
Mercury & Fluorine, that pair, might be more characteristic of island nations...Fluorine occurs naturally in water, more in water loving people...Mercury might be geologically specific to Australia(yes, the volcanic rock Australia is built upon, has much natural Mercury), although possibly a tendency of the peoples that are able to live there, since violence also comes with excellent physical stamina...(Think athletes)...This is all speculative & not a generalization at all...Further study is needed...(been trying to see tendency by race, location, climate, country...a delicate pursuit at best)! :)

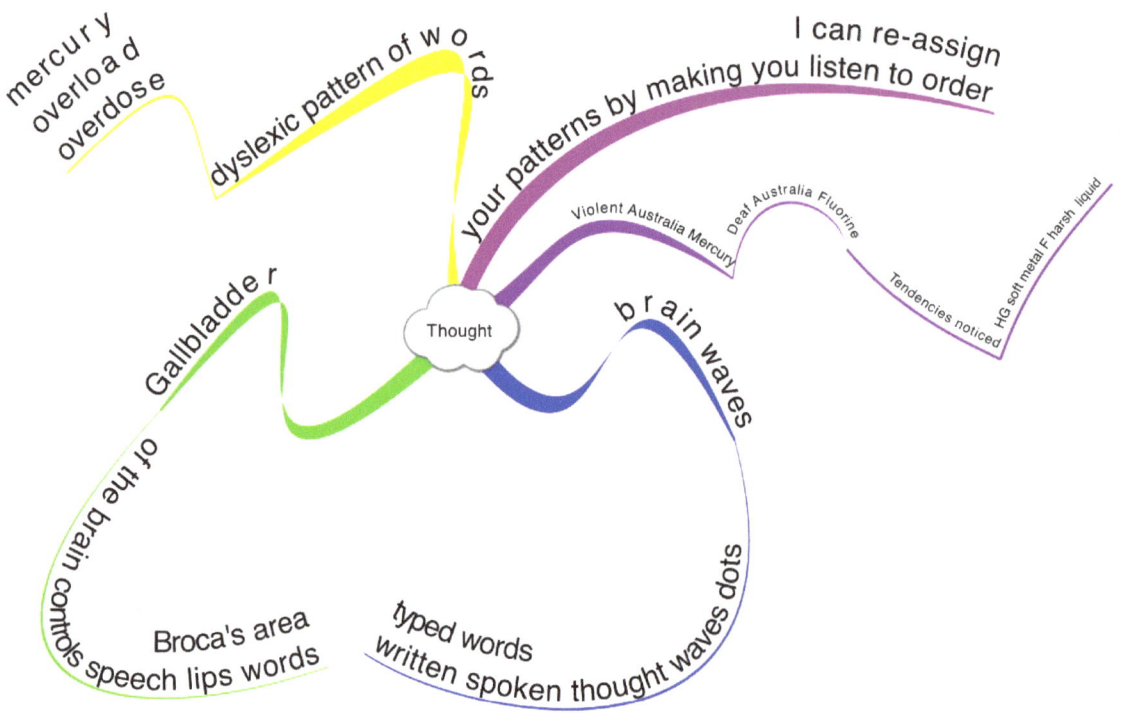

Elements:where to find,

Gallbladder-

Magnesium (a Minus Element): Dolomite Rocks, Zeolite rocks, Epsom Salts oral or topical for bathing, Pill
separator substance used around pills to make them not stick together often found in completely strange places like drugs that are supposed to build bone or vitamins that are supposed to build cartilage...Living in Ontario, Canada means you live on a Dolomite magnesium bedrock...Sometimes just choosing a location with the geology you need is the right decision!
*Palmated larkspur(staphysagria), an herbal, is also a Magnesium, as is Lavender...

Gallbladder:

Mercury (a Plus Element):Burnt Poop Fume(really) from sewage treatment plants (people who live near water(Boston,Florida, California, Lake
Ontario-you will notice personality differences in friends who live near water- high mercury makes people violent, aggressive, & they will argue something even if they are in the wrong, this is mercury buildup in the gallbladder), often have very elevated mercury levels-but it is not always a bad thing-they may have some communication problems but their cartilage development is fantastic!), Rudraksha Beads(these are an amazing red mercury seed that comes strung on copper wire or other wire & you wear them & the mercury makes your arthritis feel better-from India usually-often from monks
there-they will bless them for you too if you are lucky!), Parad Malas(this is a mercury bead mixed with silver), bacon, Kishka(intestines- cooked with stuffing & gravy), Hot dog casings, Salt, Haggis, Blood Pudding, Pepperoni...Again-Salt is a cheap & easy way to Raise bilirubin levels in the gallbladder...(only for those with magnesium in excess btw)...Bacon...Salt... Hypernatremia means too much salt in the body...I have put salt, sodium chloride NaCl in the Mercury Hg section...because sodium chloride salt acts like mercury just in a lesser way...They act alike...Gallbladder
Mercury makes you colder...(even though you Think you will feel hotter)

Yes SALT falls into the MERCURY category, but just less...

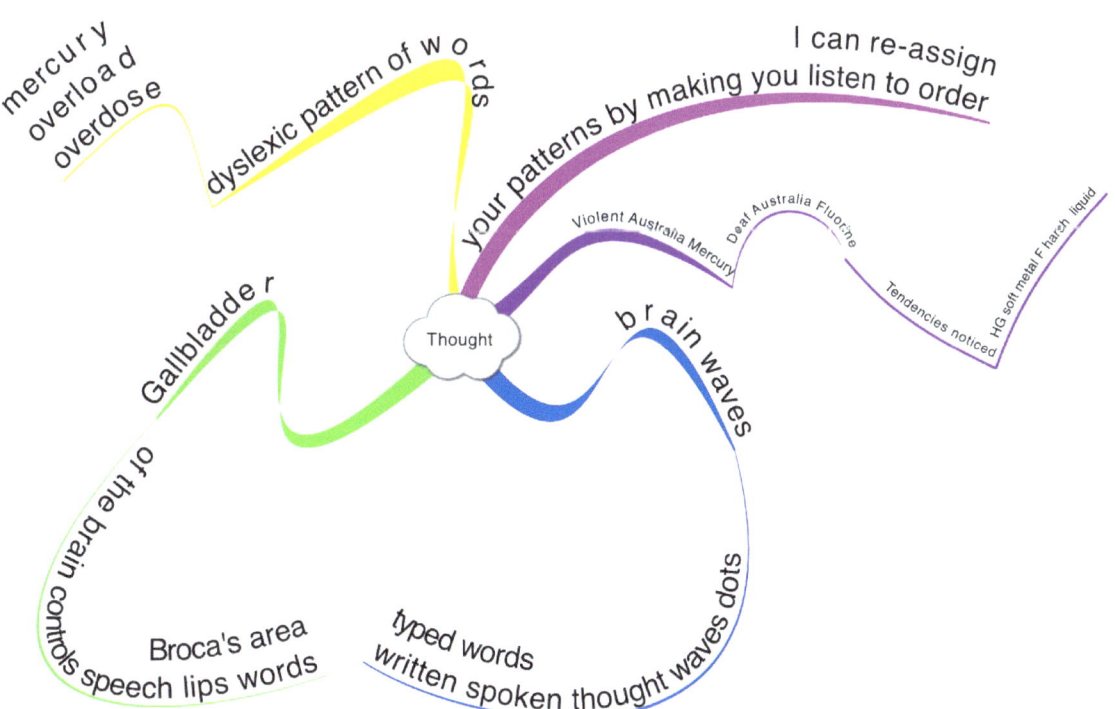

Also Mercury occurs naturally in volcanoes...If you live near a volcano, you get this rich cartilage building Mercury...An active volcano spits Mercury out as a fume...Mercury from other people's active volcanoes can enter the water, & when that water flows to your country, you can absorb that in your skin from water contact...Volcanic rock contains Mercury...

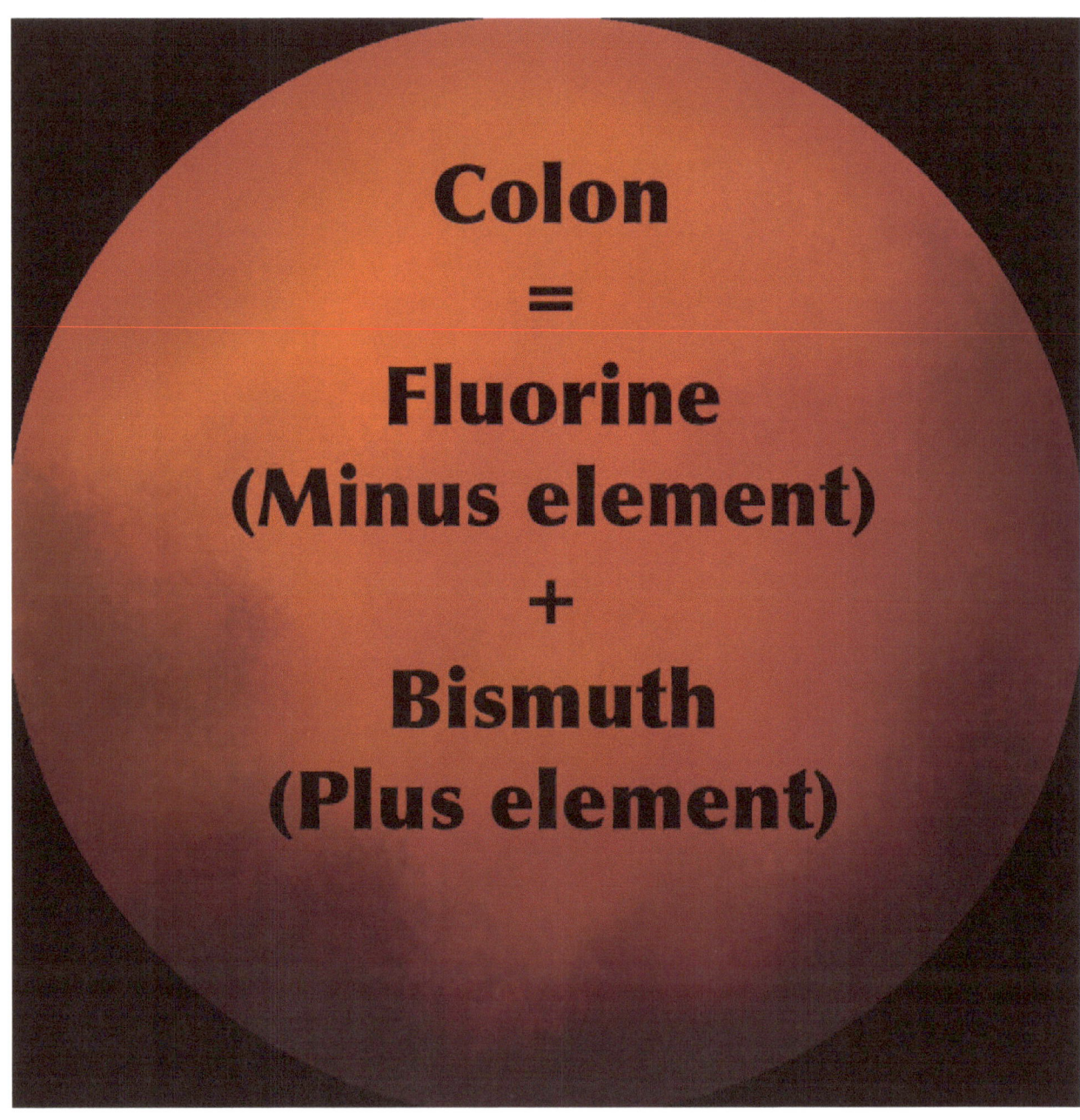

Colon=Fluorine(Minus element)+Bismuth(Plus element)

http://www.grovecanada.com/blog/2013/10/the-temporal-lobe-the-ears-the-colon.html

Heroin is a Fluorine element...The new Alternative injectable is called GcMAF & is very similar to Heroin, I think...

Melatonin is an Indium element which is related to the Bismuth family but stronger...

fluorine excess hearing loss epilepsy ALS

left temporal is plus side(Bismuth)

Bismuth Plus element (also Indium & melatonin)

Temporal Lobe to Colon to Bismuth Plus to Fluorine Minus

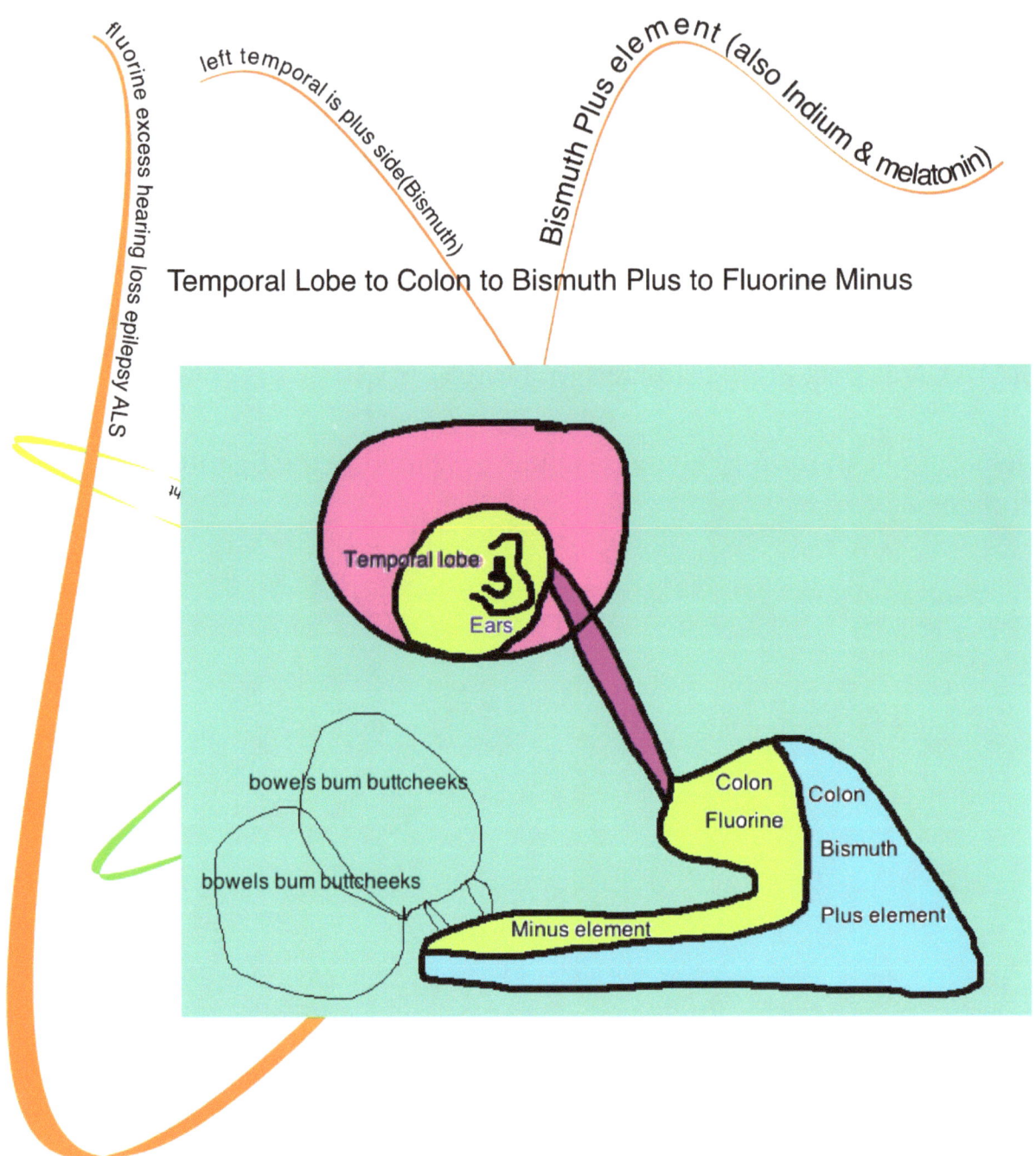

So the Colon addresses the Temporal Lobe...Within that temporal lobe there are some specific areas that handle specific things...Two big ones within the Temporal lobe are the PINEAL gland which handles falling asleep & waking up, or darkness & lightness, or Melatonin/Bismuth/ Indium & Fluorine...The other big one is WERNICKE's area, which handles Understanding speech(which is to be differentiated by Broca's Area, the gallbladder brain part, which handles PRODUCING speech & connects to the mouth & lips)...

  Now within Wernicke's area, inside the temporal Lobe, following our PLus element theory at the LEFT side of the brain, & Minus element theory to the right side of the brain, then, also, the left side of Wernicke's area, the PLUS element side, handles DOMINANT thought understanding type things like stereotypes or cliches or iconic things like the Easter bunny likes chocolate or Cavemen carried clubs or Ice cream is sweet...

The right side of the brain in Wernicke's area handles understanding of NON-dominant type thoughts like understanding poetry, or abstract art, or quirky music that is non-traditional or philosophy that is new & different...

In Broca's area, with autism, a Mercury type excess, lack of speech might be noticeable, since Broca's area handles speaking...

In Wernicke's area, if there is a Bismuth excess(damage or environmental suffocation like say from coal mining activity), then there is speech but it can be nonsensical...Why maybe? Because if the dominant side, the Plus element side(the left hemisphere of), the Bismuth side of Wernicke's area is all gunked up with Bismuth(say coal char particulate airborne from burning wood fires), then aphasia might occur, which is real words, but put together without the filter of understanding of what you are saying...Aphasia might be a sign that someone has taken too many anti-epileptic drugs(Bismuth) & needs to back off...

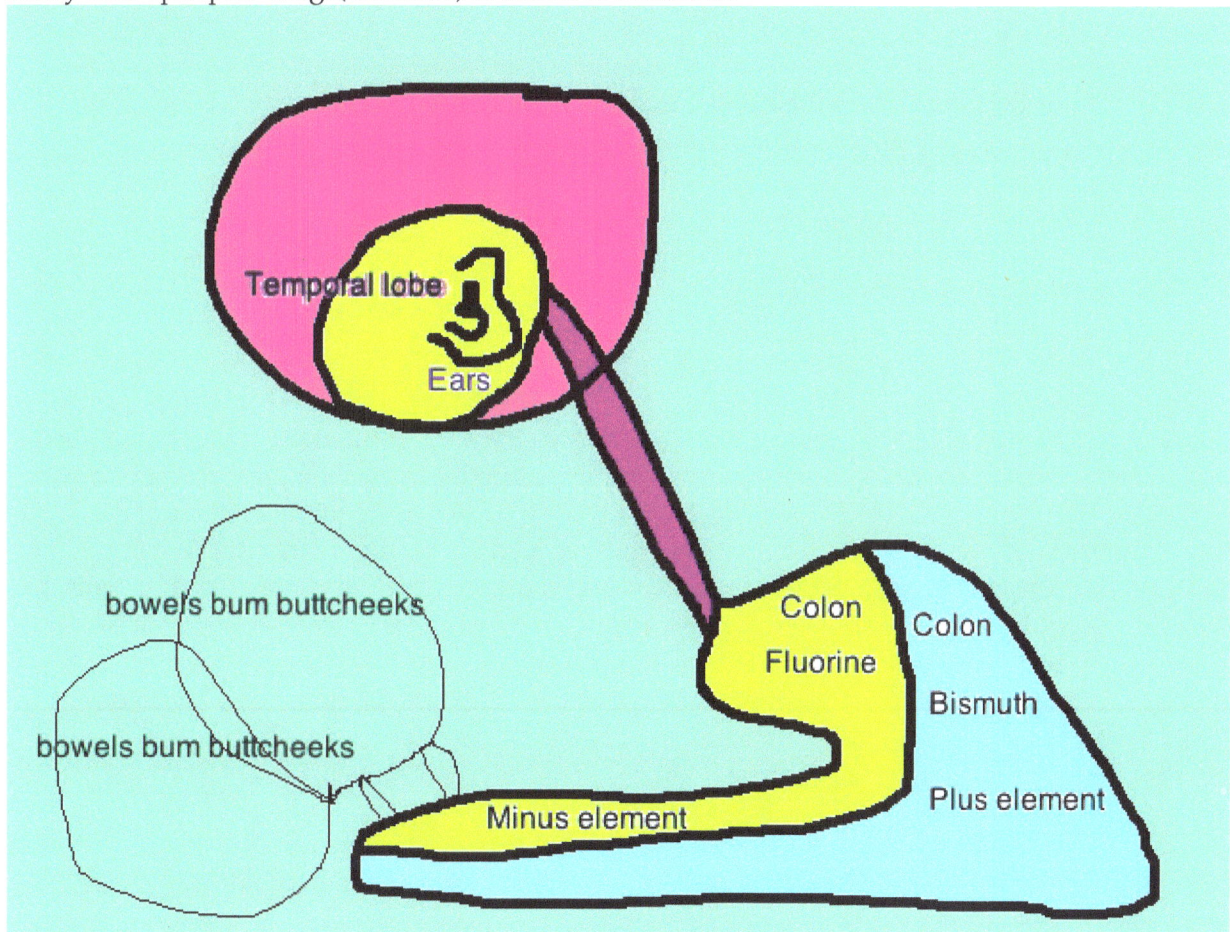

Colon:

Too much Fluorine (a Minus Element): Paralysis, Can't move, Crohn's disease,Diarrhea, Fabry an 'Orphan' illness, domesticity(used on prisoner's of war to tame 'wildness'), Sweaty-ness, discoloured teeth due to fluorosis, hearing loss...also vision loss...Epilepsy...Seizures...

Gulf War syndrome(gulf war soldiers were exposed to fluorine gas/sarin which is a high dose of fluorine-they have experienced epilepsy, Lou Gehrig's disease, slow paralysis, seizures-which all confirm that fluorine is the trigger to epilepsy & ALS Amyolotrophic Lateral Sclerosis(Lou Gehrig's)

-did you know Lou Gehrig's father had epilepsy?
  A further confirmation of the direct link between fluoride(athletes consume large amounts of water that has both natural & artificial fluoride inside), ALS & epilepsy...

Fluoride causes diarrhea, paralysis, it is an anesthetic, & also causes domesticity in terms of behaviours, the severe diarrhea & loss of nutrient can lead to hearing loss as well as seizures & epilepsy...It appears that Scottish people or of Scot ancestry are most vulnerable to fluorosis which means excess fluorine...Epilepsy...Lou Gehrig's disease...ALS...Seizures...Amyolotrophic Lateral Sclerosis...

Tetanus Typhus Seizures ...Are all Fluorine, fluorine added to the body...(the killed virus or bacteria is a fluorine type of virus bacterium)...

Tetanus vaccine seizures Ottawa: Note...The tetanus shot has been LEGALLY correlated to epilepsy, even if symptoms appear 6 years later...(Is this actually the cause of the Gulf War soldiers' epilepsy & Lou Gehrig's?)

In the case of Gulf War veterans who now have Lou Gehrig's & Epilepsy maybe it was a 4 pronged trigger to selectively attack one group of soldiers...Like this:1)Weaker immune system (those with)2)Got a TETANUS shot(or shot containing tetanus & diptheria & other killed virus bacterium)3)Were exposed to fluorine gas when they exploded those biological warfare factories in the Gulf(fluorine gas is SARIN gas)4)Were the type of person to drink huge amounts of fluoridated waterSo those 4 selection criteria were the soldiers who got Fluorine excess ailments like epilepsy & ALS Lou Gehrig's...Note:Wild Indigo Root tea contains Indium(Indium is its own element on the periodic table of elements-it is common for stronger doses of the same thing to get their own name) a Bismuth type element which antidotes fluorine but way stronger...It helps you sleep better & is an anti-seizure tea if you take more...(start with one teaspoon of the wild indigo root herb in a cup of boiled water, steep for 10 minutes, strain(we use the Bodum coffee maker thing to strain our tea leaves-you put the leaves in then steep then squish the press down-easy)...

Landau Kleffner Syndrome=Fluorine excess(epilepsy is a sign you are in a fluorine excess area)...

Colon:
Too much Bismuth (a Plus Element): Severe Constipation...(very dangerous actually)...Severe

constipation which can trigger a whole host of problems throughout the body...Organ damage...Toxin build-up...

Indium is also very much like Bismuth , just way stronger...Indium is found in melatonin...Indium is also found in the heroin recovery drug ibogaine...Too much Indium can cause wild weird hallucinations & dreams & nightmares, but also can cause the sensation of wanting to vomit, & then, actual vomiting...Indium in the form of Melatonin has been very helpful to people with ALS Amyolotrophic Lateral Sclerosis-which makes sense, since Melatonin falls into the Bismuth category which antidotes fluorine on our chart, & ALS is a Fluorine excess imbalance...(Hearing Loss & Crohn's disease & Insomnia & Epilepsy & Double Vascular arch & vascular ring(these are distended heart disorders), would also then respond well to Melatonin, them being all Fluorine excess imbalances as well)...

Grove Body Part Chart is always a work in progress...

Elements:where to find,

Colon-

Fluorine (a Minus Element): Fluoride, drinking water in urban areas,
toothpaste, the GHB drug is fluoride the date rape drug, Anaesthetics are all fluorine, Propfyl the thing Michael Jackson took is fluorine, It's a paralytic, Fluorosis which is fluorine poisoning actually causes discolored teeth!

 Fluorine is found naturally in shellfish-My mum had a conch(a mollusk) salad at the Mutiny hotel(the whirlpool was closed because they were shooting a Playboy centrefold, & the hotel room had a mirror on the ceiling above the bed) in Florida, & later got so sick & diarrhea too-Conch in the warm soft waters of Florida can have huge amounts of natural fluorine in it...

 The warmer & softer the water, the more fluorine...Hard water means it has minerals in it like Calcium which offset the minus effect of fluorine...People with Cystic Fibrosis(An Aluminum excess) tend to be more immune to cholera(cholera is a Fluorine excess disease with lots of diarrhea)...
****Fluoridation of Calgary's (province of Alberta, country of Canada) water stopped in May 2011.

***A type of pufferfish with spiny urchin like prongs, has within those prongs, a heavy duty concentrated fluorine, which causes paralysis, & mimics death in those who take it...Think Romeo & Juliet...(plots where death needs to be mimicked)...

See the Gallbladder section for my new notes on Polio which I had mistakenly put there first...I now think Poliomyelitis is a Fluorine excess problem due to the paralytic effect which is characteristic of Fluorine excess problems, as well as the esophageal problems which also go with fluorine excess problems...

Colon:

Bismuth (a Plus Element): Activated Charcoal Pills, Burnt wood, Coal, Charcoal (I Like activated charcoal pills for Crohn's disease & Fabry- but you need to take like 6 charcoal pills or equivalent in powder form a day to make it really work)...

Note:The element called INDIUM acts just like Bismuth but is WAY stronger...Wild Indigo Root contains Indium otherwise known as Baptisia Australis(there are other names too)...

Dilantin, which as a generic drug is called Phenytoin, is also in the Bismuth category of elements, like Indium, & melatonin...Dilantin is another anti-epileptic...How do we know it resembles Melatonin for instance? Both substances have wild weird dreaming as a side effect, as does Indium, & Bismuth in high enough doses...All make you pukey if too much is taken...All have anti-epileptic properties, just some stronger than others...The herbal Wild Indigo root is a cheaper, over the counter way of getting the same stuff...All these things mitigate fluorine in the Colon...

http://www.herbs2000.com/herbs/herbs_wild_indigo.htm This link has alot of information that is maybe too much, but some of it is good...To be noted, a concoction using wild indigo root (Indium/Bismuth) plus echinacea(an aluminum) & white cedar(a Nitrogen) & a repeat of echinacea but another kind(another aluminum element)-it's a 4 herb thing...This concoction has been used as RECOVERY after taking antibiotics(a selenium thing)...
  So after an antibiotic round, the 4 herb thing they mention in the link-is good for replenishing the body...*I also like wild indigo root for insomnia, epilepsy, ALS, & Crohn's disease...
  ***It HAS been used for Crohn's disease, on the record by the way...

*my father, a neuro-ophthalmological surgeon once told me of a village where everyone was dying but doctors didn't know the cause...They researched & tested to no avail...Finally they just started giving the people water, because the severe diarrhea was causing dehydration...Everyone got
better...Sometimes you just need to treat the symptoms!

  In Crohn's & Fabry, diarrhea is the biggest issue...You can die from diarrhea... Bismuth, activated charcoal pills, will stop the diarrhea(or just use Pepto Bismol for the Bismuth, but know that it also contains Titanium which is like aspirin & can cause memory loss & also ringing in the ears) & balance out the fluorosis in the colon...My feeling about these two problems is that fluoridation is the trigger...It appears that urban areas have more fluoride in the water than rural areas...Know that...

Also: Epilepsy,

Tourette's & Seizures are associated with excess Fluorine in the Colon, treat the same way-with Bismuth...(also withdraw from all fluoride sources)...

Colon: Fluorine Excess: I'd also add to this list, Myotonic Dystrophy & the concurrent enlargement of heart sometimes complicated by a Double Aortic Arch...I would hasten to add that fluoridated water causes this excess, in particular, to people who tend to drink large amounts of water...(Also, now the TETANUS SHOT HAS BEEN CORRELATED TO EPILEPSY & OTHER FLUORINE EXCESS DISORDERS I HAVE MENTIONED HERE)...

Colon: Too much Fluorine: ALS Amyotrophic Lateral Sclerosis (lou Gehrig's disease) Gulf war veterans were exposed to Fluorine gas & now many have ALS...Which explains succinctly that ALS is Fluorine excess...Note that Motor Neuron disease like ALS can also come with seizures like epilepsy, which is also fluorine excess...(activated charcoal powder antidotes fluorine btw) (The element Indium acts like Bismuth charcoal but is much much stronger...It is a stronger antidote that corrects fluorine imbalance, suppresses epileptic seizures, & allows one who is insomniac to sleep deeper...)

I'd like also to mention the element called Indium...Indium acts like Bismuth but is much much stronger...Indium metallicum has been used in Germany to treat epilepsy...Since epilepsy is a fluorine excess & Bismuth is its antidote, then Indium, which acts like Bismuth logically works in theory, but also in studies, in practice as a remedy for epilepsy...

Indium supplements or liquids should also work then towards ALS Lou Gehrig's & Crohn's...Indium is rare & would be dangerous to anyone not suffering from a fluorine related excess...because it would constipate, like Bismuth does...

Also: (Note Angelman's Syndrome is an epilepsy category ailment as well)...Wild Indigo Root is documented for controlling seizures...It contains the right antidoting element to fluorine-the Indium element as well...Indium is like Bismuth but stronger...Same effect though-controls seizures, makes you sleep better, stops the diarrhea associated with excess fluorine, thereby allowing the body to keep its own nutrients...

See my blog post about epilepsy, Lou Gehrig's, Angelman's syndrome, ALS (all fluorine poisoning ailments), here http://www.grovecanada.com/blog/2013/09/i-wrote-to-the-teen-in-ottawa-who-needs-help-nowhere-are-my-facebook-comments.html

Comment regarding marijuana as a treatment for epilepsy:

"The article implies that there is marijuana or surgery...In fact epilepsy has been controlled in numerous other ways...Raising salt levels, either in the diet or by taking salt tabs, has controlled epilepsy...The homeopathic element Indium metallicum(indium is also in supplements) controls seizures...The plant called Wild Indigo Root prevents seizures...The article should be less biased towards marijuana as a treatment for children, since the long term side effect of marijuana is severe memory loss, which is unfortunate in a child who is building life long memories...As well, marijuana is not a new treatment...This is misleading...Withdrawing from all fluorine sources is also a path...Gulf War veterans exposed to sarin gas (a fluorine gas) came home with Lou Gehrig's disease & epilepsy...Which now gives us a very strong correlation between fluorine levels & epilepsy...This might allow parents to remove all traces of fluorine from the child's life...The cause being removed is even more powerful than treatments...No?"

Big Cause: Ok, so besides fluoride in the water supply in Ottawa, how are children there getting a fluorine overdose?
Ok, well, the answer is a bit sad...
At two months old, Ottawa protocol says that children must get some sort of a tetanus shot...
It is tetanus with usually two other things, but tetanus is the big one...
Why? because It has been shown that the tetanus shot, after being given to children, causes 3 times as many children to have a seizure...Than those who did not get the tetanus shot...(You can read about that statistic at http://www.WDDTY.com if you search for epilepsy & tetanus in their search engine)...
   It is a known possible side effect, adverse effect of the tetanus shot...Seizures...Guillain-Barre syndrome is another adverse effect...Guillain-Barre resembles Lou Gehrig's disease...
   You see Tetanus is a disease like Typhus & Cholera...It is a fluorine excess illness...Same effects as induced fluorine, but you get it from cutting your skin or drinking bad water & it gets inside...
   So, a killed tetanus sample in a vaccine, might, perhaps in a warmer weather, or the refrigerator wasn't that cold or something in the lab, that Tetanus might create a problem in a young child (two months old is the protocol remember)...
   Fluorine is worse in warm waters...Also in soft water with less minerals...So on a warm day, in a child who might be low in minerals, that tetanus shot could induce a fluorine excess, causing a seizure, or even a seizure disorder...
   I happen to know about that tetanus shot effect...Unfortunately...I was at Harvard University, & I cut my shin on a bike pedal, the way that always happens when you miss the pedal & it swipes back at you to bite your shin...
   It was enough of a three pronged messy cut that I went to the student hospital...So they gave me a Tetanus shot immediately...
   Then I got really sick...Really really sick...Not only that I had no idea what was wrong with me...High fever, disoriented...
   A friend from Norway got me a refund, & put me on a plane back to Toronto...The cold Toronto air corrected my problem almost right away...
   One wonders if this global warming trend, is causing children in Ottawa to show ailments that are more characteristic of hotter weather children?
   The tetanus shot seems to be, like fluorine itself, far more active in a warm climate than in a cold one...
   At any rate, the tetanus shot may be the cause of this new rash of young children in Ottawa with epilepsy disorders...

Which also makes one wonder, how many soldiers before going out to the Gulf War in 1991 got a Tetanus shot? Was their epilepsy from the Sarin gas(fluorine gas) or from the Tetanus shot itself(also a fluorine based illness)?

http://www.ageofautism.com/2011/01/us-vaccine-court-rules-routine-dtap-diptheria-tetanus-pertussis-shot-legal-cause-of-epilepsy-death.html

Yes epilepsy is definitely correlated to the TETANUS shot, even if symptoms only appear after 6 years...(after getting the tetanus shot)...http://www.coping-with-epilepsy.com/forums/f22/vaccine-related-seizures-2607/

http://forums.webmd.com/3/epilepsy-exchange/forum/1357 Even an adult whose epilepsy is under control(seizure free) can have that re-triggered by getting a Tetanus shot...

- See more at: http://www.grovecanada.com/blog/2013/09/i-wrote-to-the-teen-in-ottawa-who-needs-help-nowhere-are-my-facebook-comments.html#sthash.WmjnxlIk.dpuf

The water in this neighbourhood is over-fluoridated...

Over-fluoridation causes diarrhea, insomnia, sometimes hearing loss, thinning teeth & later brown spots on your teeth...It can also cause seizure & later epilepsy...Lou Gehrig's disease, a slow paralysis as well...Fluoride causes repression of wildness behaviours & domestic behaviours enhanced...Fluoride was used on prisoners of war to make sure they did not rebel...Fluoride is in the GHB rape drug, Propofyl the anaesthetic that killed Michael Jackson, & regular anaesthetics...Also Sarin Gas that was deployed during the Gulf War in the early 1990s is fluorine...

The two things that antidote Fluorine are:Bismuth(activated charcoal pills or powder), Indium(a rare element that mimics Bismuth but is stronger)...Indium is found in supplements that contain Indium (see Amazon just type in Indium to find supplements liquids or pills)...Indium is found in Indium metallicum an homeopathic remedy...

Indium is also found in a plant called Wild Indigo Root...You can buy a bag of Wild Indigo Root from Herbies Herbs on Queen street, which is on the North side, between Spadina & bathurst street...It is not expensive for a large bag of herb...Take the herb, like a teaspoon & steep it into some boiled water...Drink before bedtime...It will help you sleep deeper, & you will feel more settled & refreshed when you wake up...Use judiciously, it is strong...You can also drop the herb into your tap water...It will clear out the excess fluoride...

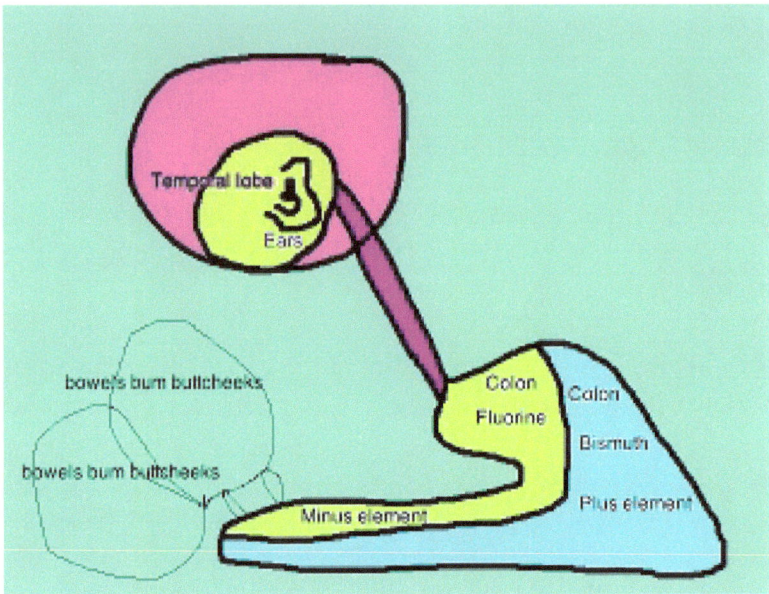

A Comment I wrote in response to a slam on herbals:Wild Indigo Root contains the rare element called Indium on the Periodic Table of Elements...Indium has been in used in German medicine to quiet epileptic seizures...This flower has a lesser amount of Indium, so it is safer as an anti-insomniac & to increase deep sleep & REM stages...There are direct correlations to fluorine & epilepsy, as well as Lou Gehrig's...I have also been looking into the same correlation between fluorine & heart irregularity(Double Aortic Arch) at birth...I assure the previous commenter, that, addressing a deficiency by providing the element that is lacking, through a very modern solution, that can be made into a tea, titrated for a child, & bought readily, is about as modern as modern medicine gets...The future of medicine is in solutions that are precise & easy to take & obtain...I made no mention of discarding any other courses of treatment either...Most modern pharmaceuticals are based on herbs...It would be ignorant to ignore a better answer, for something that may be unaffordable, not easy to take or swallow, & imprecise in its efficacy...Titration is so important with children...Drug level drugs are so much more dangerous...The same herbal format can be taken or withdrawn, in a much easier way, depending on effect...

Melatonin is also a Bismuth/Indium/Charcoal type thing...Melatonin makes Parkinson's disease worse(*Phosphorus is in the Spleen, excess Phosphorus is Parkinson's, think mold, but Melatonin, being also a Plus element, though in the Colon not in the Spleen, can block the Colon up, not allowing Phosphorus to excrete from the Spleen...)

 ****Ibogaine from the Iboga root is a Bismuth/Indium/Charcoal , to the highest degree-causes intense dreaming like Melatonin another Charcoal/Bismuth/Indium, but way more...
 Ibogaine also can induce ataxia a Parkinsonian-LIKE
 (meaning not exactly the same thing)
 symptom where you cannot walk...(It is used to detox from heroin, as seen on the tv show *Homeland)...

(a LACK of Charcoal/Bismuth/Indium/Melatonin element, makes you sleepless, paralyzed, too domestic, not rebellious, not wild, tame, thin teeth, diarrhea tendency, epileptic or seizure prone, in higher deficit ALS, Amyolotrophic Lateral Sclerosis, Hearing Loss, Deafness, paralysis slow or fast(you can also get raped easier when you lack the Bismuth family of elements)...

Dyes often fall into the Bismuth category...Like the red dye they get from cockroaches to colour food...Indigo Carmine I think it's called...Blue dyes too...They made the heads of flowers fall off...Oh I told you that already...Just again, in case people tell you dyes are all safe...I know about dye dangers because I used to drink Shirley Temples, with red dye number 5 in the maraschino cherry(which I hated anyway, nothing so fluorescent I thought could be safe to eat-I just like the Seven-up & the sweetness & that I could have a cocktail too like a grown-up instead of tap water which was icky & little pieces floated in it)...They banned that red dye...But I see it sometimes, & they just changed the number...(just don't eat anything that is glowing unless you are a glow worm predator or maybe a firefly-ok I take that back-I am sure that red dye is probably nutritious for someone who is lacking in glowingness, please forgive my intrusion)...

Sari

End of the Basic Chart sections, beginning of more freeform thoughts, brain parts, more complicated stuff:

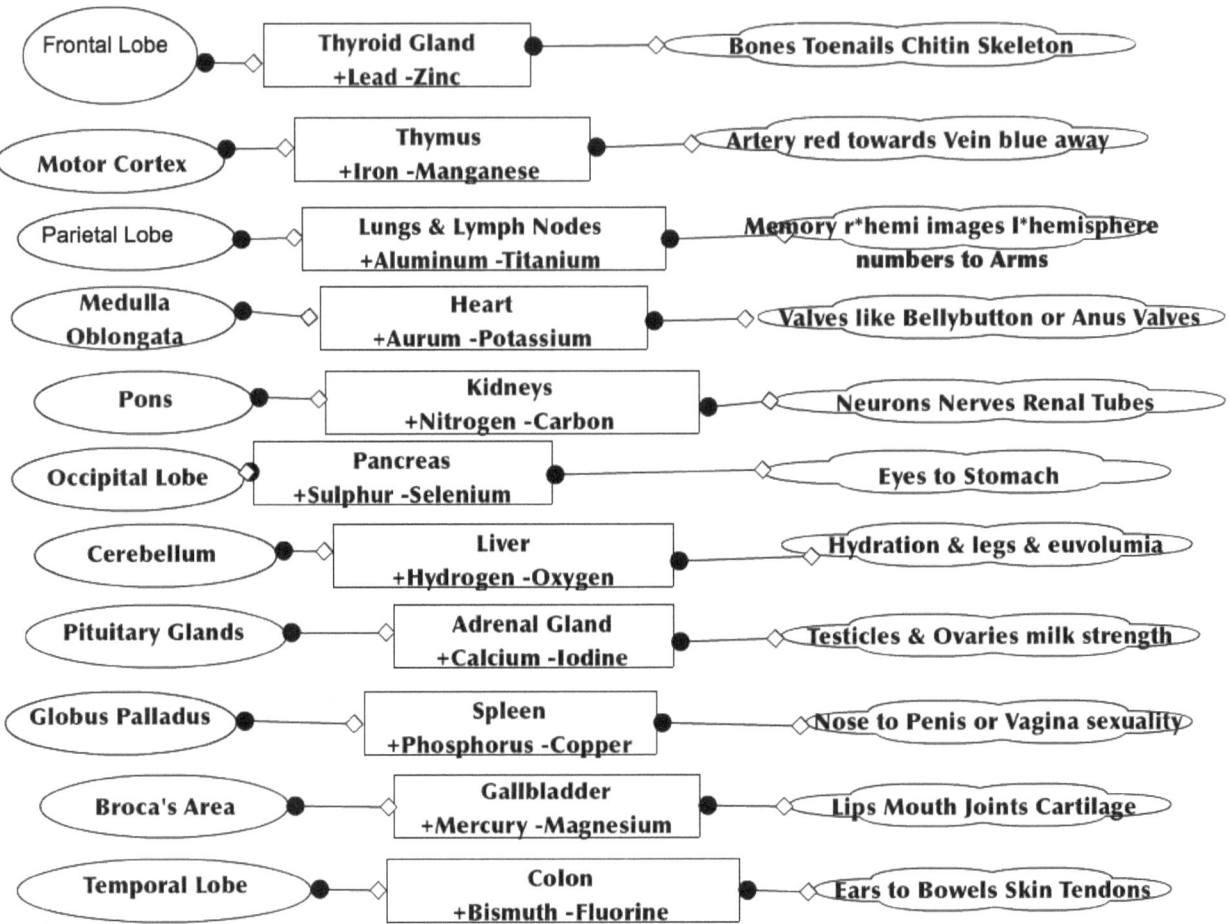

Above is a new chart...Shows brain, body, limb connections...In order...!

Oct.23, 2013, Wednesday:

My app is at Fun e-books in the iTunes store...(it is a teeny version-abbreviated alot)

It is a free e-book called Grove Body Part Chart

It is based on a print book called Grove Body Part Chart:A Medical Arts Innovation

By teaching people how to heal themselves, they won't have to drive so much because they can walk...

healthy people walk more, drive less...

That is my app...

(Note:My app is found when searching for Fun E-Books in the iTunes store, But it is part of a gathering of other people's books as well...Just look for Grove Body Part Chart to see my own app within that app...It's an app within an app...Sorry it costs more to have a standalone app...)

Sari Grove

p.s.I wrote the book so this all my own copyright...

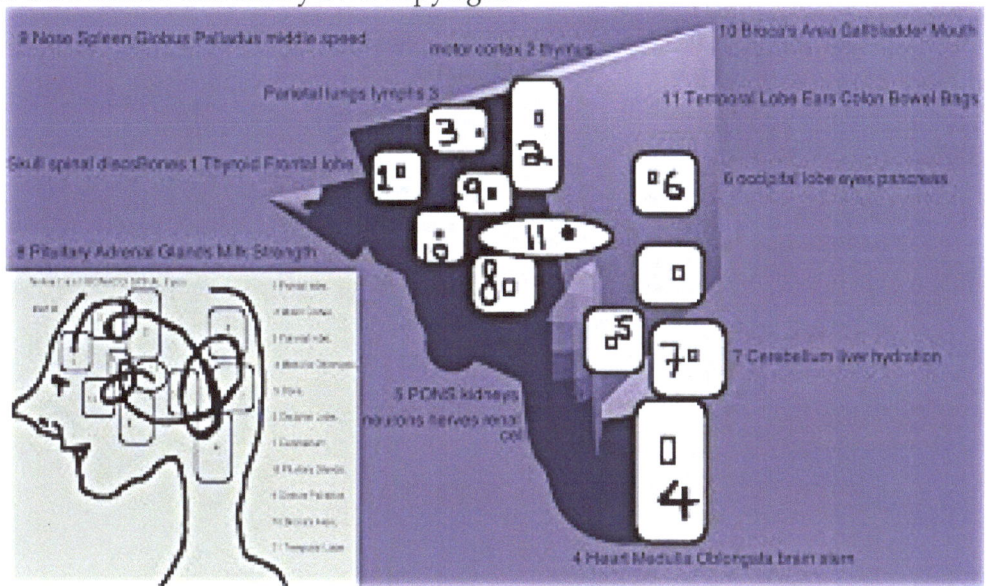

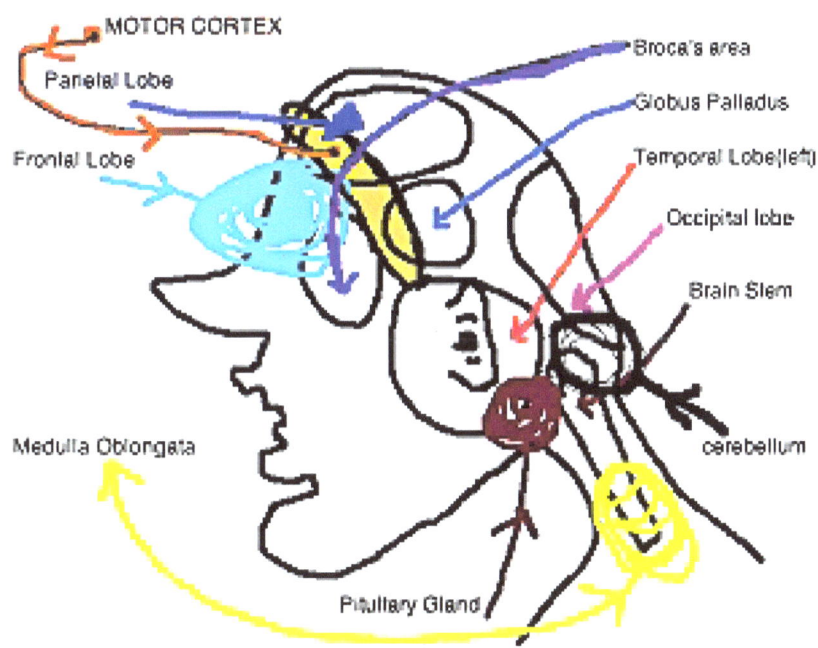

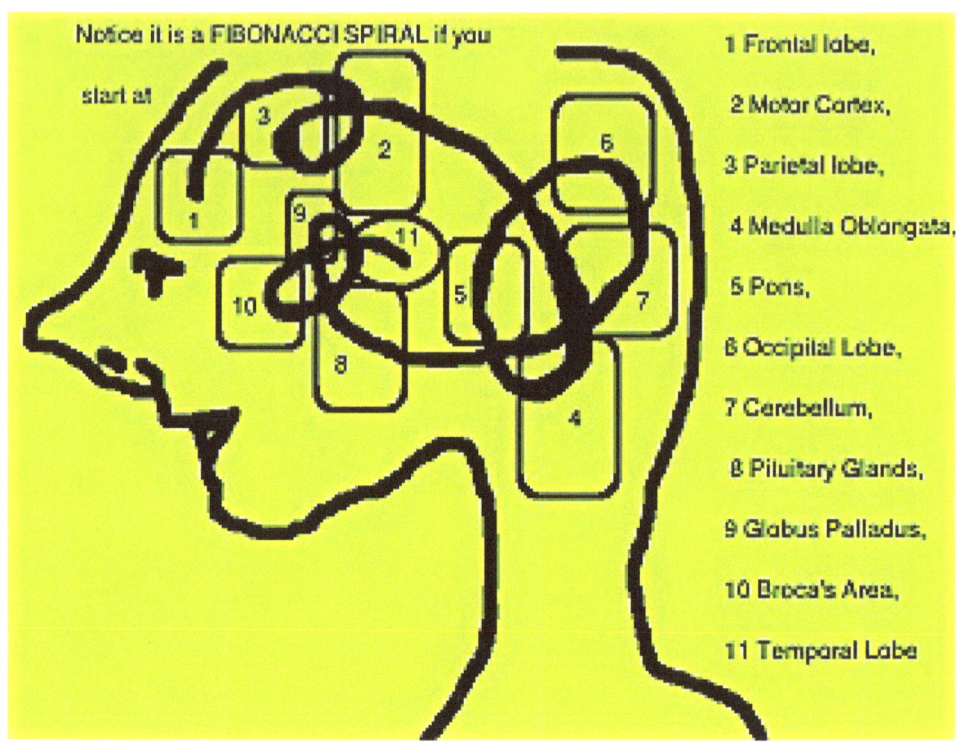

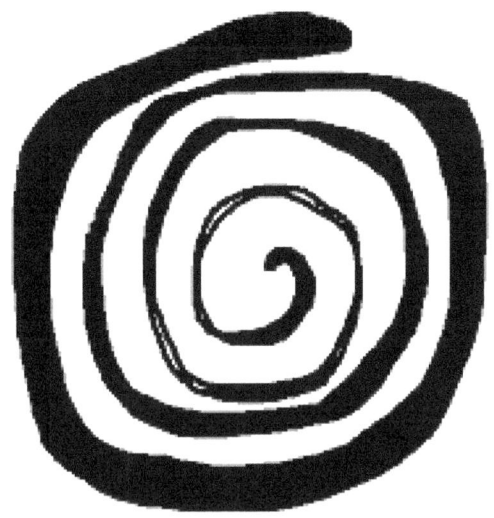

Notice it is a FIBONACCI SPIRAL if you

start at

1 Frontal lobe,

2 Motor Cortex,

3 Parietal lobe,

4 Medulla Oblongata,

5 Pons,

6 Occipital Lobe,

7 Cerebellum,

8 Pituitary Glands,

9 Globus Palladus,

10 Broca's Area,

11 Temporal Lobe

This is the book description you might see online when you go to buy the paperback version of this book...

The brain part connects to the body part...

(sing to the tune of "the kneebone connects to the,

thighbone, the thighbone connects to the,

hipbone,

the hipbone connects to the, ...)

The Frontal lobe connects to the Thyroid gland, the

Motor Cortex connects to the Thymus gland,

The Parietal Lobe connects to the Lungs & Lymph Nodes...

Note on Sidedness:

The LEFT side of the Frontal Lobe is a Plus element dominant LEAD (Plomb) side...

The Right side of the Frontal Lobe is a Minus Element Zinc side...(hemisphere...)

The Parietal Lobe also follows this same pattern, of

Left side is Plus dominant Aluminum,

Right Parietal is Minus element Titanium dominant...

So, if brain parts are LEFT side Plus element(see my Books for plus minus element list)...

Then ARE body parts the reverse, yes, probably...(or True?)

Let's see: Body Parts...

If reverse(because cross switch theory that brain side is opposite to body side, ie:left side of brain controls right body part side, then...)

So the RIGHT hand is LEAD dominant, because the LEFT side of the Frontal lobe is Lead dominant

(plus element)...

The left hand is then Zinc dominant...

The right lung is then Aluminum dominant...(Like the left side of the Parietal lobe)

The left lung is them Titanium dominant...

We know lefties then are Minus element dominant, since Minus elements in the brain are on the right side of the brain...

We know right handed people then are Plus element dominant since the left side of the brain is Plus element dominant...

We know lefties tend to be more artistic, because the left side of the body, & the right side of the brain, in the Parietal lobe is the image or drawing side...sides...

Righthanded people tend to be more numerical or logical since the left side of the Parietal lobe for example handles numbers & math & logic...

Are women more Minus element dominant & men more Plus element dominant?

Not sure, but interesting to think about...There is definitely an inclination to think so...But that could be my own bias...

Grove Body Part Chart

Organ	Minus	Plus
Thyroid	Zinc	Lead
Thymus	Manganese	Iron
Lung & Lymph Nodes	Titanium	Aluminum
Heart	Potassium	Aurum
Kidneys	Carbon	Nitrogen
Pancreas	Selenium	Sulphur
Liver	Oxygen	Hydrogen
Adrenal Gland	Iodine	Calcium
Spleen	Copper	Phosphorus
Gallbladder	Magnesium	Mercury
Colon	Fluorine	Bismuth

Thyroid Frontal lobe bones toenails chitin...

Thymus Motor Cortex Artery red towards Veins blue away...

Lungs & Lymph Nodes Parietal Lobe arms memory right hemisphere images left hemisphere numbers...

Heart Medulla Oblongata Connectors- brain stem to body stem ie: bellybutton valve to anus valve ...

Grove Body Part Chart

Organ	Minus Element	Plus Element
Thyroid	Zinc	Lead
Thymus	Manganese	Iron
Lung & Lymph Nodes	Titanium	Aluminum
Heart	Potassium	Aurum
Kidneys	Carbon	Nitrogen
Pancreas	Selenium	Sulphur
Liver	Oxygen	Hydrogen
Adrenal Gland	Iodine	Calcium
Spleen	Copper	Phosphorus
Gallbladder	Magnesium	Mercury
Colon	Fluorine	Bismuth

Kidneys "Pons"(think Ponds) sits at the top of the brain stem creates cells renal tubes neurons nerves, a line is just a bunch of dots holding hands...

Pancreas Eyes Occipital Lobe Stomach...bag...

Liver Cerebellum Hydration legs volume...

Grove Body Part Chart

Organ	Minus Element	Plus Element
Thyroid	Zinc	Lead
Thymus	Manganese	Iron
Lung & Lymph Nodes	Titanium	Aluminum
Heart	Potassium	Aurum
Kidneys	Carbon	Nitrogen
Pancreas	Selenium	Sulphur
Liver	Oxygen	Hydrogen
Adrenal Gland	Iodine	Calcium
Spleen	Copper	Phosphorus
Gallbladder	Magnesium	Mercury
Colon	Fluorine	Bismuth

Adrenal Gland Pituitary Gland "balls" ovaries seaweed hair milk. Mass.

...

Spleen Nose Globus Palladus Penis
(vagina womb room uterus)...

Gallbladder, Broca's Area in the brain, Cartilage bendy-ness joints (corpus Coloseum)the stuff that lines the outside of your hockey helmets' like... The outer 'lining' of your skull...

*(The inner lining Phosphorus muck see spleen page)...

Grove Body Part Chart

Organ	Minus Element	Plus Element
Thyroid	Zinc	Lead
Thymus	Manganese	Iron
Lung & Lymph Nodes	Titanium	Aluminum
Heart	Potassium	Aurum
Kidneys	Carbon	Nitrogen
Pancreas	Selenium	Sulphur
Liver	Oxygen	Hydrogen
Adrenal Gland	Iodine	Calcium
Spleen	Copper	Phosphorus
Gallbladder	Magnesium	Mercury
Colon	Fluorine	Bismuth

Colon, Temporal Lobe, Ears, Balance, Bowels, Bum, Buttcheeks, Bags, containers, where things go, garbage disposal... **(Storage hold, Insurance policy, savings & holdings)

Grove Body Part Chart

Organ	Minus Element	Plus Element
Thyroid	Zinc	Lead
Thymus	Manganese	Iron
Lung & Lymph Nodes	Titanium	Aluminum
Heart	Potassium	Aurum
Kidneys	Carbon	Nitrogen
Pancreas	Selenium	Sulphur
Liver	Oxygen	Hydrogen
Adrenal Gland	Iodine	Calcium
Spleen	Copper	Phosphorus
Gallbladder	Magnesium	Mercury
Colon	Fluorine	Bismuth

Organ	Minus Element	Plus element
Thyroid	Zinc	Lead
Thymus	Manganese	Iron
Lungs & Lymph Nodes	Titanium	Aluminum
Heart	Potassium	Aurum
Kidneys	Carbon	Nitrogen
Pancreas	Selenium	Sulphur
Liver	Oxygen	Hydrogen
Adrenal Gland	Iodine	Calcium
Spleen	Copper	Phosphorus
Gallbladder	Magnesium	Mercury
Colon	Fluorine	Bismuth
Organ	Minus Element	Plus Element

Grove Body Part Chart: Research

Organ	Minus Element	Plus element
Thyroid	Zinc	Lead
Thymus	Manganese	Iron
Lungs & Lymph Nodes	Titanium	Aluminum
Heart	Potassium	Aurum
Kidneys	Carbon	Nitrogen
Pancreas	Selenium	Sulphur
Liver	Oxygen	Hydrogen
Adrenal Gland	Iodine	Calcium
Spleen	Copper	Phosphorus
Gallbladder	Magnesium	Mercury
Colon	Fluorine	Bismuth
Organ	Minus Element	Plus Element

Top of body to bottom: Minus elements get stronger & Plus elements get weaker... Inside body, to Outside parts...ie: Lead is in bone, a building block, whereas Bismuth is in a tendon, an outer detail part...

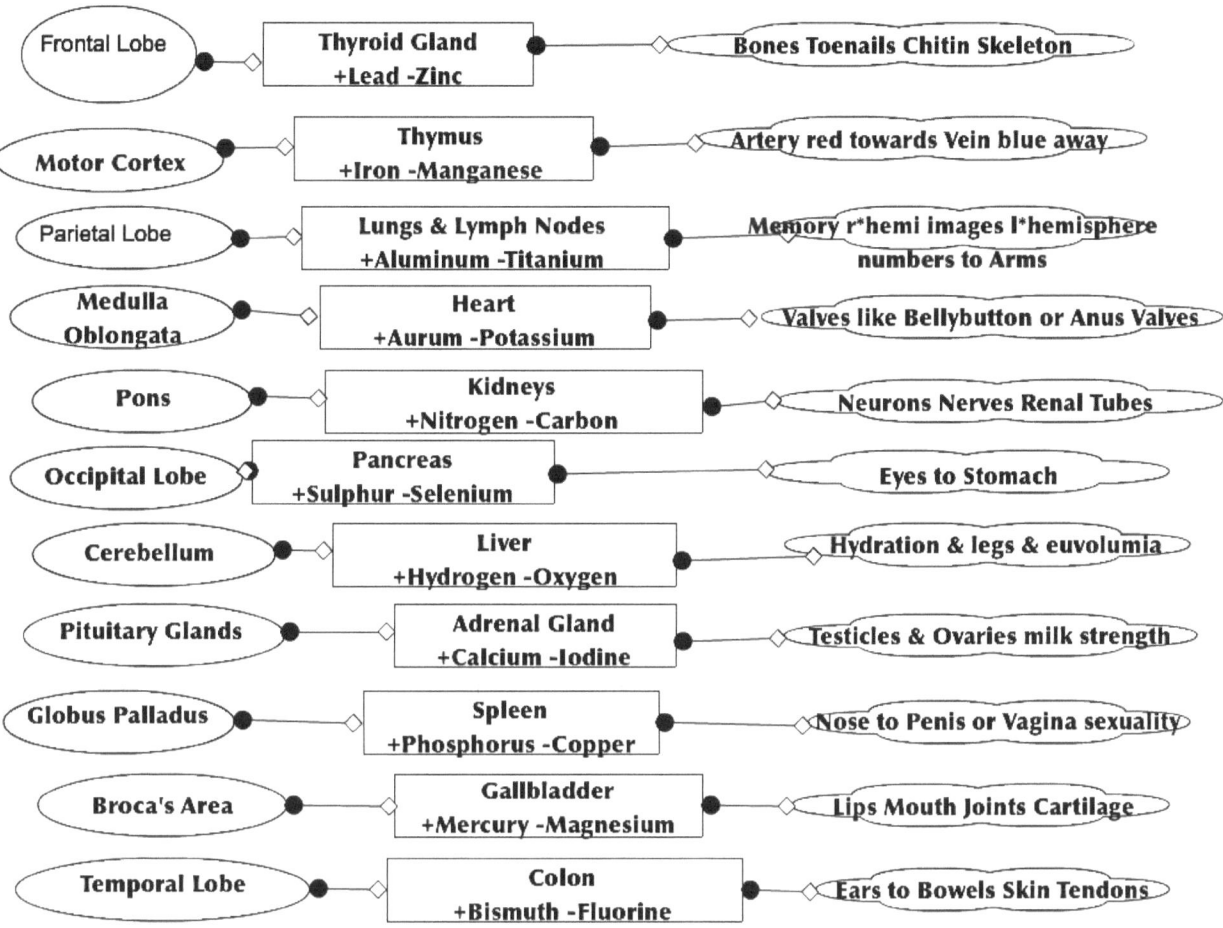

Frontal Lobe	Thyroid Gland +Lead -Zinc	Bones Toenails Chitin Skeleton
Motor Cortex	Thymus +Iron -Manganese	Artery red towards Vein blue away
Parietal Lobe	Lungs & Lymph Nodes +Aluminum -Titanium	Memory r*hemi images l*hemisphere numbers to Arms
Medulla Oblongata	Heart +Aurum -Potassium	Valves like Bellybutton or Anus Valves
Pons	Kidneys +Nitrogen -Carbon	Neurons Nerves Renal Tubes
Occipital Lobe	Pancreas +Sulphur -Selenium	Eyes to Stomach
Cerebellum	Liver +Hydrogen -Oxygen	Hydration & legs & euvolumia
Pituitary Glands	Adrenal Gland +Calcium -Iodine	Testicles & Ovaries milk strength
Globus Palladus	Spleen +Phosphorus -Copper	Nose to Penis or Vagina sexuality
Broca's Area	Gallbladder +Mercury -Magnesium	Lips Mouth Joints Cartilage
Temporal Lobe	Colon +Bismuth -Fluorine	Ears to Bowels Skin Tendons

Grove Body Part Chart

Organ	Minus Element	Plus Element
Thyroid	Zinc	Lead
Thymus	Manganese	Iron
Lung & Lymph Nodes	Titanium	Aluminum
Heart	Potassium	Aurum
Kidneys	Carbon	Nitrogen
Pancreas	Selenium	Sulphur
Liver	Oxygen	Hydrogen
Adrenal Gland	Iodine	Calcium
Spleen	Copper	Phosphorus
Gallbladder	Magnesium	Mercury
Colon	Fluorine	Bismuth

Grove Body Part Chart: Research

Organ	Minus Element	Plus element	Duty
Thyroid	Zinc	Lead	Bones
Thymus	Manganese	Iron	Blood white & red
Lungs & Lymph Nodes	Titanium	Aluminum	Muscle dark & white, eggs, spermatozoa
Heart	Potassium	Aurum	Seals & Valves
Kidneys	Carbon	Nitrogen	Neurons & Nerves & Renal Tubes
Pancreas	Selenium	Sulphur	Lumps, Filler, Holes like bellybuttons
Liver	Oxygen	Hydrogen	saliva, water, oxygen
Adrenal Gland	Iodine	Calcium	Milk breast milk boobs
Spleen	Copper	Phosphorus	semen, puss, snot, lube
Gallbladder	Magnesium	Mercury	cartilage elbow knee jaw shoulder ankle
Colon	Fluorine	Bismuth	Tendons inner fibrous skin & outer skin
Organ	Minus Element	Plus Element	Duty

The Yx Yx Yx designation in the globus palladus is the male...
In the Thymus...Yx...
In the gallbladder...Yx...

If the person is a female, the order in the cavebrain would be Xy, not Yx...
& in the Thymus Xy...
& in the gallbladder Xy...

Take the Yx...Reverse the Order to Xy...Take the y molecule...Reverse the y stem by folding it back, the stem of the letter y...Then move it to the right, your right as you are viewing this page...This will form an x letter...The female is merely an Xx...A folded back y gene...But the second x is smaller than the first X... or you could say the male gene Y is merely an extended x gene, but bigger than the x...
For the Y gene to become an x gene, the x gene must APPEAR smaller...It is really the same amount, but looks smaller, even on a computer screen...

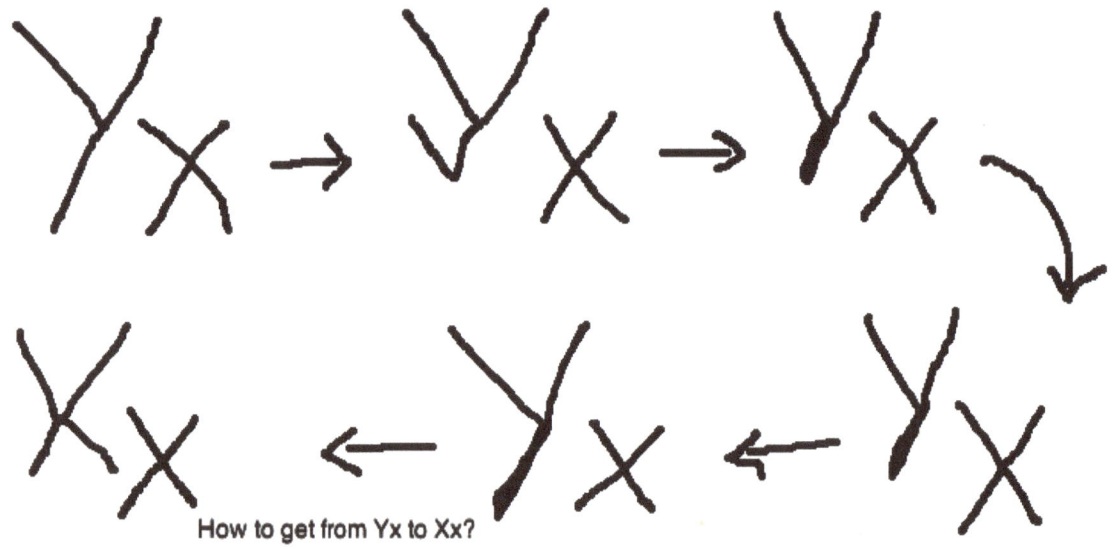

How to get from Yx to Xx?

Fold the stem of the Y gene...

Then grow a leg to the viewer's right, or

the molecule's left...The person's

left...Posit:Are women lefty tendency???

Alfre Woodard:"[on her marriage] We were both taught, "You pick your friends on how they treat you - not by what they have or what they look like". We get twice the cultures."

Alfre Woodard:"I've surrendered to Facebook just to maintain a relationship with my children. I also follow them on Twitter. They're witty, irreverent, hip. I have only eight friends. Otherwise, it becomes a job.

Additional Thoughts on Nothing in Particular:

http://www.fluoride-class-action.com/fibromyalgia-or-skeletal-fluorosis-aliss is it fibromyalgia or is it skeletal fluorosis or chronic fluoride poisoning? (hint: Fibromyalgia is a mercury deficit, whilst skeletal fluorosis or chronic fluorine poisoning is a *Bismuth(or **Indium) deficit...

Comment:Elements on the Periodic Table of the Elements are often very similar, in the same family, just that one is weaker & one is stronger...Like an herbal remedy is the same thing as a drug just the herbal is weaker...

Charcoal, Bismuth & Indium all act the same way, but Indium is much much stronger...The herbal form is in Wild Indigo Root, which contains Indium...Indium the metal is stronger than that herbal & can be worn against the skin...It is an anti-epileptic, an anti-insomniac, & reverses fluoride poisoning...

Put a tea thimble full of wild indigo root into a pitcher of tap water & leave overnight in the fridge...It balances out artificially fluoridated water...Better than charcoal/Bismuth...

Note: Lead(PLOMB) is a lesser form of LITHIUM...Builds bones...(same family)...

Some florists are allowing flowers to drink water that contains blue dye in it...The heads of the flower then turn blue...It is a very unusual effect...I was given a bunch of these very unusual flowers...Several days later, the heads of the flowers all fell off...The blue dye was too heavy...heavier than just plain water...I would put Blue Dye into the Bismuth/Indium/ Charcoal/serotonin/Melatonin category in the Colon organ...I write this as a warning to people who get dyes injected into their bodies...From tattoos to dyes for medical tests be forewarned that dyes can be dangerous...Hair dyes...Make-up dyes...Theoretically, Fluorine is the antidote for dyes, in the Colon...As you know fluorine is found in toothpastes & in large bodies of water, naturally...Dentists use way too much fluorine including the gas form...So be aware...Know the elements, know the organ involved, know the antidote, then use it if need be...Some fine young genius once said:"Herbs don't work if you don't take them"...That is true! (It also holds true for drugs, exercise methods, nutritional solutions...)

Some Martial arts involve posing in 5 different animal shapes...Silently...The next level involves those 5 silent animal poses, but you then add 6 animal sounds...(plus one extra silent animal pose of course)...You don't really have to take a class to pose silently like an animal...Nor do you need a class to pose silently like an animal, then learn to make that animal's sound out loud...DOING IT YOURSELF is a great way to start an exercise program...

I have also been using My Thoughts for Mac, a mindmapping program to map out ideas for this book...Thank you...

Thank you also to http://www.ArtBizCoach.com for encouraging me to continue pursuing the medicine stuff when it was still more in its infancy & a little kookier than it is today...(A little kookier might be an understatement...)

Some thoughts I'd like to step on again:

If you REMOVE an organ from the left lobe of the brain, like a brain part: Then you are left with RIGHT side brain dominance of that part...Since we have said the right side of the brain is MINUS element dominant, we will say then that we will have Minus element dominance of that brain part...

ie:if I remove the left side of the Frontal lobe & that contains the Plus element Lead...Then...I have remaining the right side of the frontal lobe which is the Minus element side which will contain Zinc...I will then show a ZiNc (ZN) excess tendency, like bipolar type behaviours or talking...

(This theory is a direct reference to information about a real person named Phineas Gage...I have just pushed the facts from that case into a workable sidedness theory of brain parts...And by association, of my connection charts, the body parts that connect accordingly to that brain part...and the activity that those all parts do!)

Here's a factoid I learned today:

Quicksilver is an old name for Mercury, because it quickens...Like, makes you faster...Mercury, like the volcanic rock base Australia is built upon makes you have excellent cartilage development...(It can also make you too physical, think Olivia Newton John's "Let's Get Physical" song)...(The natural fluorine in the water there though can cause some hearing loss...& more...)

But:

Back to the sidedness theories:

DAMAGE to the organ on one side, does NOT necessarily cause dominance of the UNinjured side...

So we need to distinguish between removing an organ...

&

Damage to an organ...

Ok, what's the difference?

Well...

Damage to the Spleen for example, causes Phosphorus overload, Phosphorus excess...
Removing the Spleen, does NOT cause Phosphorus excess...It causes symptoms more
concurrent with Copper excess...

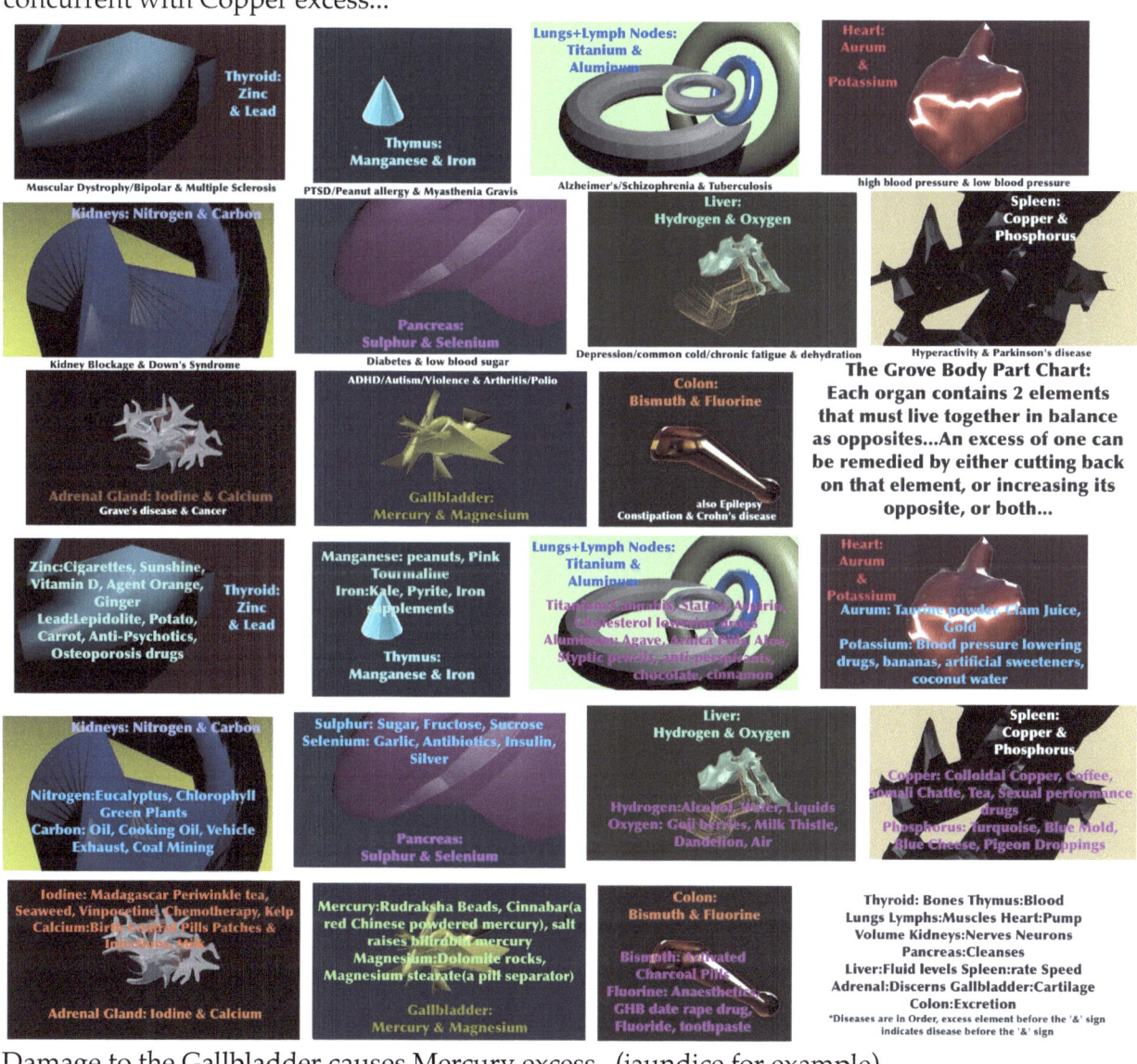

Damage to the Gallbladder causes Mercury excess...(jaundice for example)
But removing the Gallbladder causes symptoms more similar to Magnesium excess...(poohing
too much, arthritis, accidents like you break your wrist)...

So it is very important to know the difference...

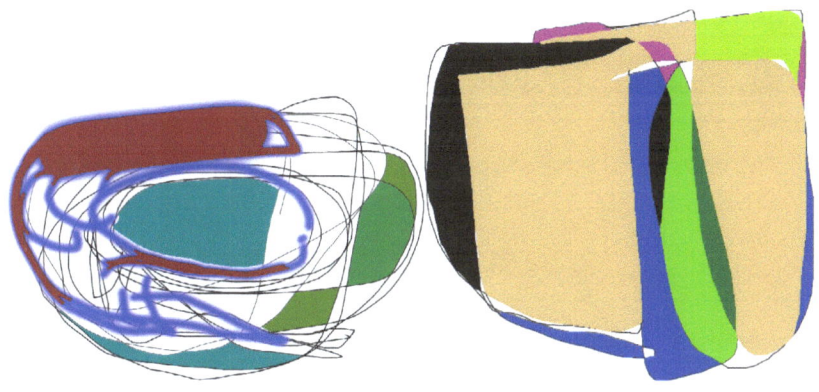

lung & lymph node	titanium	aluminum	muscle	cholesterol	One
kidneys	carbon	nitrogen	neurons	fat levels glutens	Two
spleen	copper	phosphorus tryptophan	eggs	phospholipids	Five
colon	fluorine	bismuth indium	skin	pineal gland brain? melatonin?	Seven
pancreas	selenium	sulphur	sugars	glycemic index glycolipids	Three
adrenal gland	iodine	calcium	milk	"tall" or "short"	Four
gallbladder	magnesium	mercury	tendons	fibroblast levels	Six

lung & lymph node	titanium	aluminum	muscle	cholesterol	One
kidneys	carbon	nitrogen	neurons	fat levels glutens	Two
spleen	copper	phosphorus tryptophan	eggs	phospholipids	Five
colon	fluorine	bismuth indium	skin	pineal gland brain? melatonin?	Seven
pancreas	selenium	sulphur	sugars	glycemic index glycolipids	Three
adrenal gland	iodine	calcium	milk	"tall" or "short"	Four
gallbladder	magnesium	mercury	tendons	fibroblast levels	Six

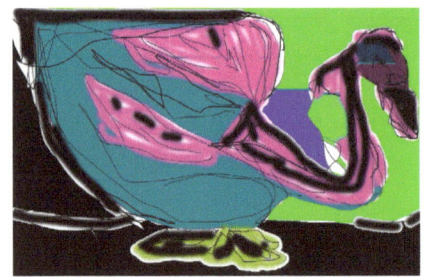

Sari Grove - your 3D viv is wowsome. love the variety of shapes, the mania, the freaky voicings, the fantasy speak, and the succinct explanation of your book's central theory. I cracked up at the character approx 6:44mins - well a few of them actually) I am intrigued by animation full stop but imagining how to do it... This to me is like the gods and godesses of the world: a mechanic fixing the car, an accountant filling in those 40 pages of gobbeldigook (that looks like a cross between icelandic and cantonese). Geniuses at work methinks. (I quiver in the corner at having to do either) . I salute you for the massive learning curve - HUGE i presume. Congratulations.

Helen Davey, musician

A review of our 3d animated film

("The award winning film based on the bestselling book")...

You can view the 10 minute animated film on our website at

http://www.grovecanada.ca ,

on our youtube channel at

http://youtube.com/grovecanada

or on our Vimeo channel at

https://vimeo.com/channels/grovecanada ...

You can hear Helen Davey sound paintings at
http://www.helendavey.com/home.html

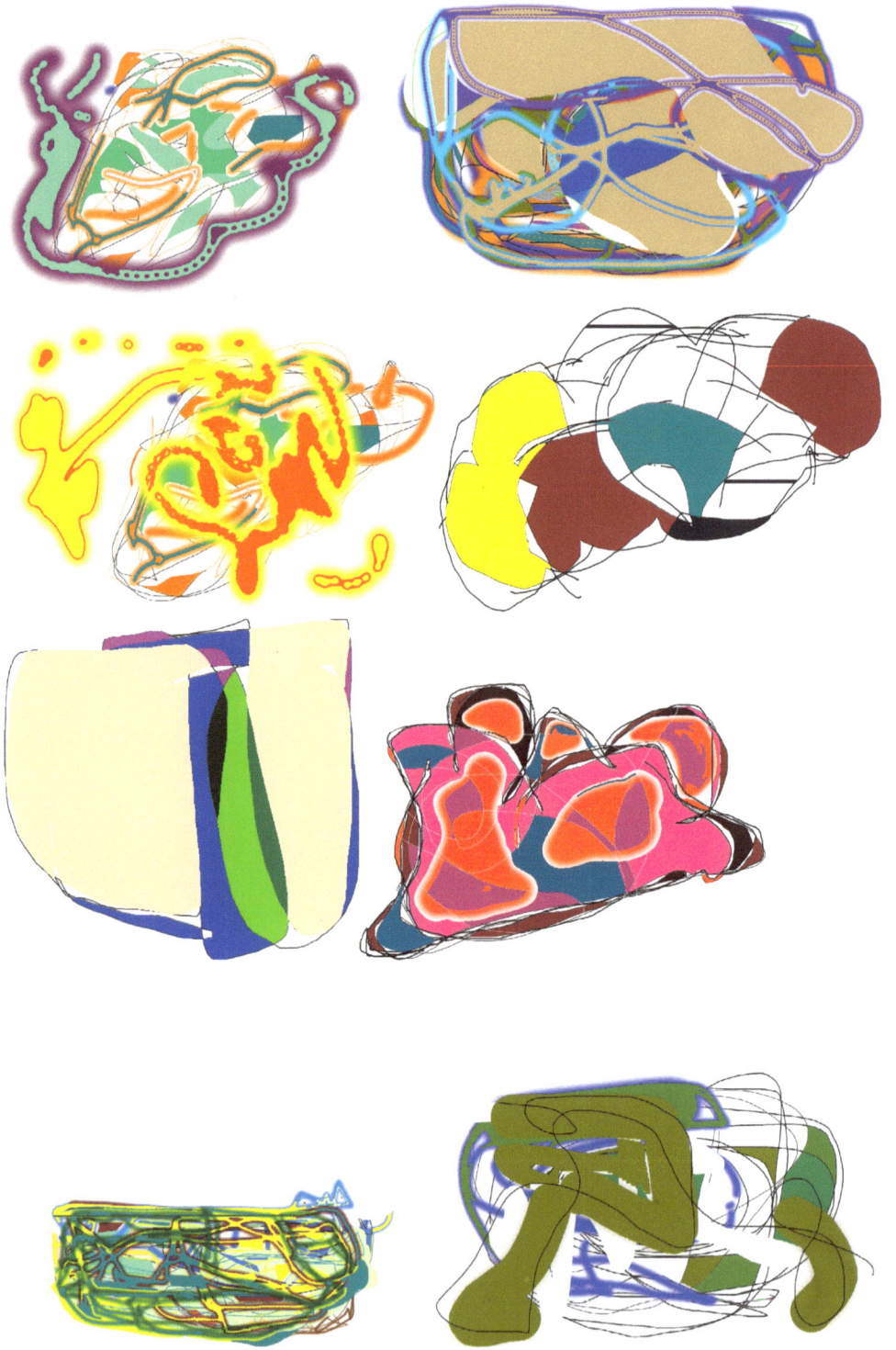

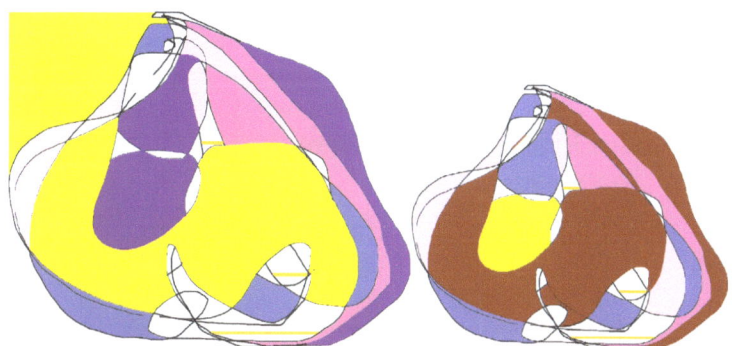

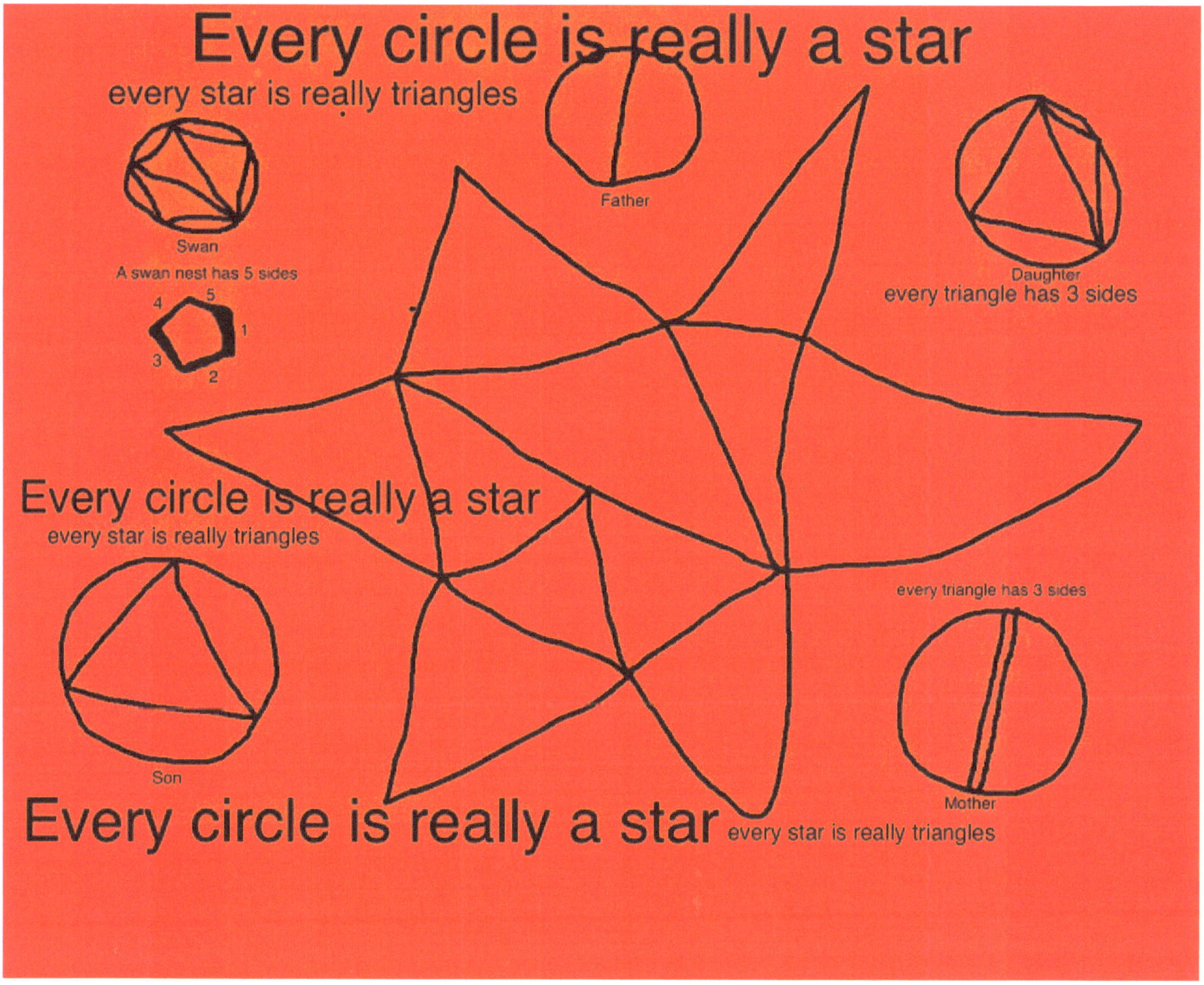

Every circle is really a star

every star is really triangles

Swan

A swan nest has 5 sides

Father

Daughter

every triangle has 3 sides

Every circle is really a star

every star is really triangles

Son

every triangle has 3 sides

Mother

Every circle is really a star

every star is really triangles

Credits:

The big orbs are Matcap materials used in Blender 3d animation software...

The MRI, PET type drawings are hand drawn with an electric mouse in the Pencil 2d animation program...

The neurology pictures are made in Paintbrush for Mac...

The ideas in this book have been come up with by Sari Grove with Joseph Grove as the wall to lean on or ask,

 & with much energy expended by professional writer Justin Wood, who inspired the neurology breakthrough...

B'Elanna Grove born Dec.1, 2004 & Jadzia Grove born April 16, 2005 are intact female bengal cats, silver & gold, from two different litters...

They provide all the eco-friendly consultation as well as the computer keyboard know-how...

(Bengal breeders tend to be very good at online programming & their kittens learn early)...

Thanks as well to all the other artists & non-artists who have been both difficult & not-so difficult...

Both types have pushed this book forward & back depending on the wind & where we needed to sail this boat to...

Please take it all with a grain of salt, as anything you read...

Sari

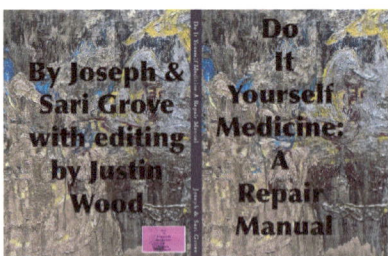

OK, SO...

I AM GOING TO SAY THIS...

THE LEFT SIDE OF THE BRAIN IS DOMINATED BY PLUS ELEMENTS...

THE RIGHT SIDE OF THE BRAIN IS DOMINATED BY MINUS ELEMENTS...

WHICH MEANS...

THAT...

THE RIGHT SIDE OF THE BODY IS DOMINATED BY PLUS ELEMENTS...

AND...

THE LEFT SIDE OF THE BODY IS DOMINATED BY MINUS ELEMENTS...

IF THERE IS ONLY ONE ORGAN LIKE THE HEART, THEN WITHIN ITS CHAMBERS, TRUE TO THE ABOVE STATEMENTS, THE RIGHT CHAMBERS SHOULD BE PLUS ELEMENT DOMINANT LIKE AURUM IS THE PLUS ELEMENT IN THE HEART...
THUS THE LEFT CHAMBERS OF THE HEART SHOULD BE MINUS DOMINANT...

IF THERE ARE TWO PARTS TO ONE ORGAN SYSTEM LIKE THE KIDNEYS, THEN THE STATEMENTS ABOVE STILL HOLD TRUE...

THE RIGHT KIDNEY WILL BE PLUS ELEMENT DOMINANT, NITROGEN...

THE LEFT KIDNEY WILL BE CARBON DOMINANT A MINUS ELEMENT...

THIS THEORY SHOULD WHOLE TRUE FOR EVERY BRAIN PART AND EVERY ORGAN AND EVERY TWO PART ORGAN SYSTEM AND EVERY ELEMENT...

I WILL CORRECT MYSELF, IF I FIND A FLAW IN THIS ARGUMENT...

(I have already corrected & updated the Kidney diagram to the PONS brain part-

(just the what side does what part not the whole thing), in this book...Please note that previous versions, our previous book, & our online blog may still have the earlier NOT updated version...)

Tags: brain, body, parts, chart, grovecanada, sari, joseph, canada, ontario, toronto, neurology, anatomy, grey's anatomy

Our MOVIE is on our Channel https://vimeo.com/channels/grovecanada at Vimeo...
The Movie is called: "The award winning film based on the bestselling book"...(It is really good & only about 10 minutes long & in High Definition!)

"Two roads diverged in a wood, and I took the one less traveled by, And that has made all the difference."
     Robert Frost

Afterthoughts:

Marfan's syndrome is Potassium excess (distended heart Aortic is key, plus long fingers, tallness)...in the Heart (Marfan's is a LOW blood pressure problem actually)...

**Marfan's is extremely low blood pressure, in the heart, which causes Aortic vessel distention (big but flaccid), as well as the long skinny fingers & the thin tallness...Low blood pressure is high Potassium, low Aurum levels(IN THE HEART which makes SEALS & VALVES)...Thus, Aurum can be boosted by taking Taurine powder, a common source...Unlike normal people, Marfan's have to raise their blood pressure to live...

Hearing Voices, Telepathy, hearing an Animal's thoughts, You are not crazy, but may have had a Concussion...

*Soundwaves are large...Thoughtwaves are smaller...Our brains are designed to hear soundwaves...When you get a concussion, your brain swells up...Sometimes you end up with a permanent swelling, edema, that stays that way...The swelling makes your brain smaller...If it makes your brain smaller anywhere near the hearing area, it affects what kind of waves you can hear...Because a concussed brain is now smaller, sometimes only the smaller thoughtwaves get through, where they did not before...So when you are very close to a person or an animal (people are animals but anyways), the smaller concussed brain can hear the tiny thoughtwaves in the other creature...if the brain heals & goes back to normal size, the larger waves come through again, & the brain is no longer able to process the tiny thought waves...Many people who were once concussed can hear the smaller thoughtwaves, but don't admit it because they think it's crazy...It's actually scientific...

(This is the Welcome Message on our New Clinical trial patient Engagement App for Mobile devices, which you can get for free by going to http://bwell.mobi/grove on Your MOBILE device-but you can also totally use it on a desktop computer, just choose HTML5 VIEW when you see the APP at the address...)

Welcome...

This is GroveBodyPartChart

the MOBILE APP...

Since this is a DIY Medicine Application, it is possible that you are having a health problem or you know someone who is...

I am very sorry to hear that...

I am here to help...

Here you will find a 23 minute VideoTalk that explains my very very basic medical chart...

Once you "get" that, you are on your way...

Book 1 is called Grove Body Part Chart:A Medical Arts Innovation...

It explains the whole chart better, & then tells you what excess or imbalance is what in which disease & where to find its opposite element, its antidote or remedy in the real world...

In the 2nd Book, called Do it Yourself Medicine:A repair Manual, I talk about some more complicated imbalances which cause diseases...

The books are full of great art done by me! because art is a great way to relax your brain from all that logical thinking(read boring thinking)...

There is a movie called RightBrain which is 10 minutes in 3d animation also done by me, which really gets your brain out of that too much thinking mode...

Which might happen from reading...

The Quizzes are fun to see if you really got the books into your head...

Plus it's a fast way to get answers,'cause if you click Submit it tells you which are the correct answers...

You can Contact me by pressing the Contact button & I totally will answer you as fast as I can...

(Be prepared, I am Canadian, so fast is like the speed of snow melting here...)

The Paperbacks button takes you to the Amazon page for my books, if you want to have a real book in your hands...

Don't feel pressured to buy...

I love trees...

My married last name is Grove & I still love Mr. Grove very much(& have been Mrs. Grove for over 17 years now!)...

You may be scared...

That's normal...

Fear is good...

It protects you from doing stupid things...

You may be around alot of doctors & nurses & technicians & they are all strangers & they all apparently want to see you naked & stick needles into you...

This is why fear is good...

You may just want to flee...

That may be a good idea...

Please don't let me be the one to tell you to ignore your fears...

They are real...

The best I can do is give you answers about medicine & health that nobody else has told you before because I hadn't thought them up yet...

With these answers you will have superpowers...

The superpower of being smarter than everyone else around you...

Now that you are going to be smarter, you will be able to make decisions about your own health, FOR YOURSELF...

It's your body, why should somebody else be the expert on it?

If you think something about something, & someone tells you you are wrong about that, because they went to this school or that school, then that makes you feel weak...

Weak is not good for your immune system or health...

I want you to know that even without reading my books or watching my videos or anything at all, that you are the EXPERT of your own body...

I don't care how crazy people say your ideas are...

It's your body & your ideas & everybody else is just wrong...

Ask alot of questions, get a second opinion, get a 3rd opinion, in fact keep getting opinions until you get one you like...

Your health is the number one thing in your life...

This is not a time to get the on sale quickie price...Beware of words like "prophylactic surgery"...

Removing parts of your body is pretty final, especially if there isn't anything wrong yet...

Genetics is a funny thing...

Your Mum could have a love of peanut butter but you can be born just alltogether hating peanuts...

So just cause a parent had one thing doesn't mean you will get it too...

Even if studies say so...

Because a genetic marker can be there & just do NOTHING at all...

Sure you might have a predisposition...

But if you figure out what that predisosition is exactly, you can STEER your boat away from that ICEBERG! I am here to help...

Help you steer your boat away from an Iceberg...

Personally I think people are taking way too many drugs & not feeding swans enough...

Personally I think that alot of new diseases are caused by all this drug taking...

I like to feed swans in winter, between November & April, because it makes me happy inside & it helps to save their lives...

I think if more people did stuff for nature, for animals & trees & fresh oxygen air, that more people would be healthy & happy...

My goal is to get people to take the power back from the so called experts including myself (which is a bit of a bind isn't it philosophically) & Do it Yourself their Medicine alot more...

Ok I'm not saying to go rogue...

I'm just saying that there are some things we can do & understand about health that might be able to be done without so much outside help...

Sari Grove, Tuesday February 4th, 2014 p.s.if you are a woman then maybe a woman doctor might be more comfortable for you...If you are 85 years old, you might prefer an 85 year old doctor...If you speak Spanish you might want a doctor who is fluent in Spanish...This is important...Don't be afraid to say:"This is what I am comfortable with & this is not"...Don't be afraid to run away...There are some scary things about medicine...If you want to run away & live in Tijuana, or Paris or Peru, then that might be a really really fun & good & healthy idea...Escape is always a fun way out...bring my books or this App...Just in case you missed something! :)

Bylaw Amendments Density:Every time a real estate developer wants to break a Bylaw density law in Toronto, they have to go to our City Council to get them to break the law & write a totally new law...

The incentive for the City Council politicians is a little know rule called Section 37...Under Section 37, if a new real estate development is seeking approvals in Toronto, 30 Per cent (%) of the EXPECTED profits from the new development have to be PAID to CITY COUNCIL...

Ok, this means that is I buy a ONE STORY house in a neighbourhood with a BYLAW DENSITY law of ONE Story houses only, then I go to City Council & say, :"Please rewrite this bylaw density law for this street because I want to build a 50 story condominium building, & I will give you 30% of the expected profits from that development, & since I expect to make 10 million dollars from that venture, I will give City Council 3 MILLION dollars to spend on whatever they want, because that is the SECTION 37 law...

So City Council says:"Ok, we will break the bylaw density law, rewrite it to make it look legal, take your 3 million dollars & approve this project which will increase density on this street by about a thousand times, & probably cause a thousand times more pedestrian vehicle collisions & casualties because bylaw density increases always do that..."

Bylaw density increases...This is why the 63 year old single mother who was taking care of her adult Down's Syndrome son, was struck down by a Mercedes van going Westbound at Spadina & Harbord streets in Toronto, & now her other son has to take over the full time caregiving of his brother...

Because the density in Toronto is illegally high for the area, for the city...Well, it would be illegal, but all the Bylaw density rules have now been rewritten for the 3 million dollars, here & the 3 million dollars there, & the 3 million dollars over there...

But all those 3 millions of dollars were supposed to go to Parks & daycares & Swans & happy things...

But it appears all that money just went into the pockets of the City Councils...

Why does it appear that way?

Because we are not seeing any new parks or daycares or schools or happy things...In Toronto...

All we are seeing is tall new buildings & tall new buildings & tall new buildings & well tall new buildings...

We are also seeing alot of people getting hit & killed by cars...(ON the other side:Wind is reduced by tall new buildings...I like wind myself , but some people are new to our cold windy country, Canada, & feel the need to suppress Mother Nature here, instead of embracing her & harnessing that energy...)

Arthur Brugger was another one of the casualties of bylaw density increases...He was struck & killed by a racing taxicab driver who was just finishing a 14 hour shift because the laws here say that taxicab drivers are allowed to operate on 14 hours shifts even though normal people must stop after 8 hour shifts...

Increased city density...Drivers working illegally long work shifts...Well, ok, the long work shifts are not illegal technically, because no one has bothered to rewrite those laws...

Sometimes health matters are not health matters at all...

Sometimes health matters have to do with politics & legal things & stuff outside the realm of a hospital or clinic or doctor's office...

Not all problems can be massaged away in an aromatherapy massage, though it is a nice way to try...

If things where you live are politically wrong then you have to speak up...

If things have happened to you that are wrong, legally, then you have to approach that health matter from more of a legal or political perspective...

Get involved...Speak out...Write about it...Tell people...Look for someone who wrote a book called DIY Law...(I am just making that up...I have no idea if that book exists yet, probably does...)

What I am saying is that you have to think outside of the box sometimes to figure out why something happened that hurt or killed you...(It can be difficult to figure stuff out, especially if they already killed you)...

Abstract ART is a great way to get your head thinking outside of the box...It teaches you that not all things are logical...(Though Spock the Vulcan would like you to believe that...Spock from Star Trek by the way)...

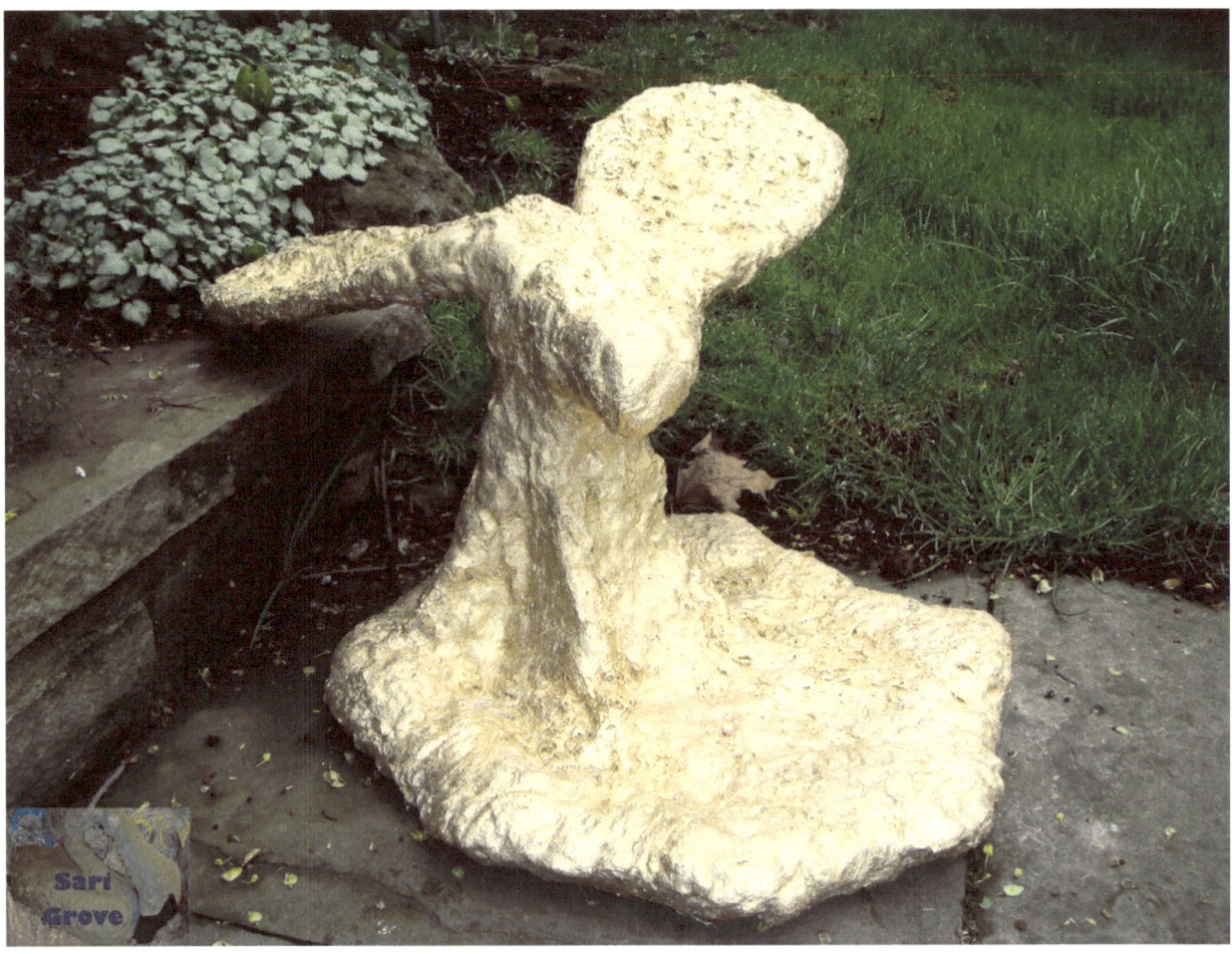

"Essence of Bee" about 2ft. x 1.5 ft x 1.5 ft. galvanized steel rods, bolts, copper strapping, aluminum mesh, covered in a custom mix of Aragonite sand, 3/4" glass fibres, white Portland cement, water, "milk", Perlite, silicate sand, with eco-friendly cement blue paint integrally mixed in, with al fresco gold powder screed in to the wet, sealed with No VOC eco-friendly concrete sealer...

Make friends with a BEE today! (I love bees)

Sari

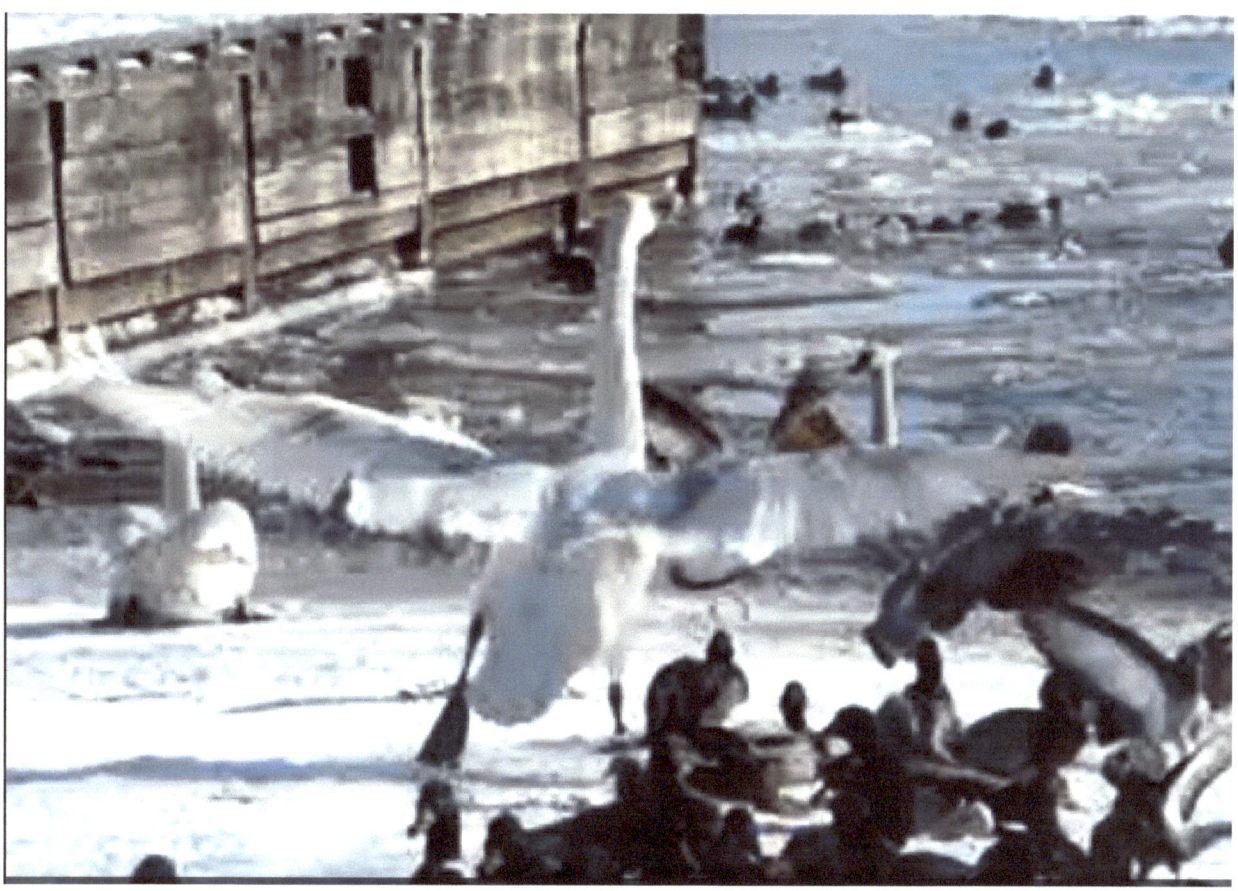

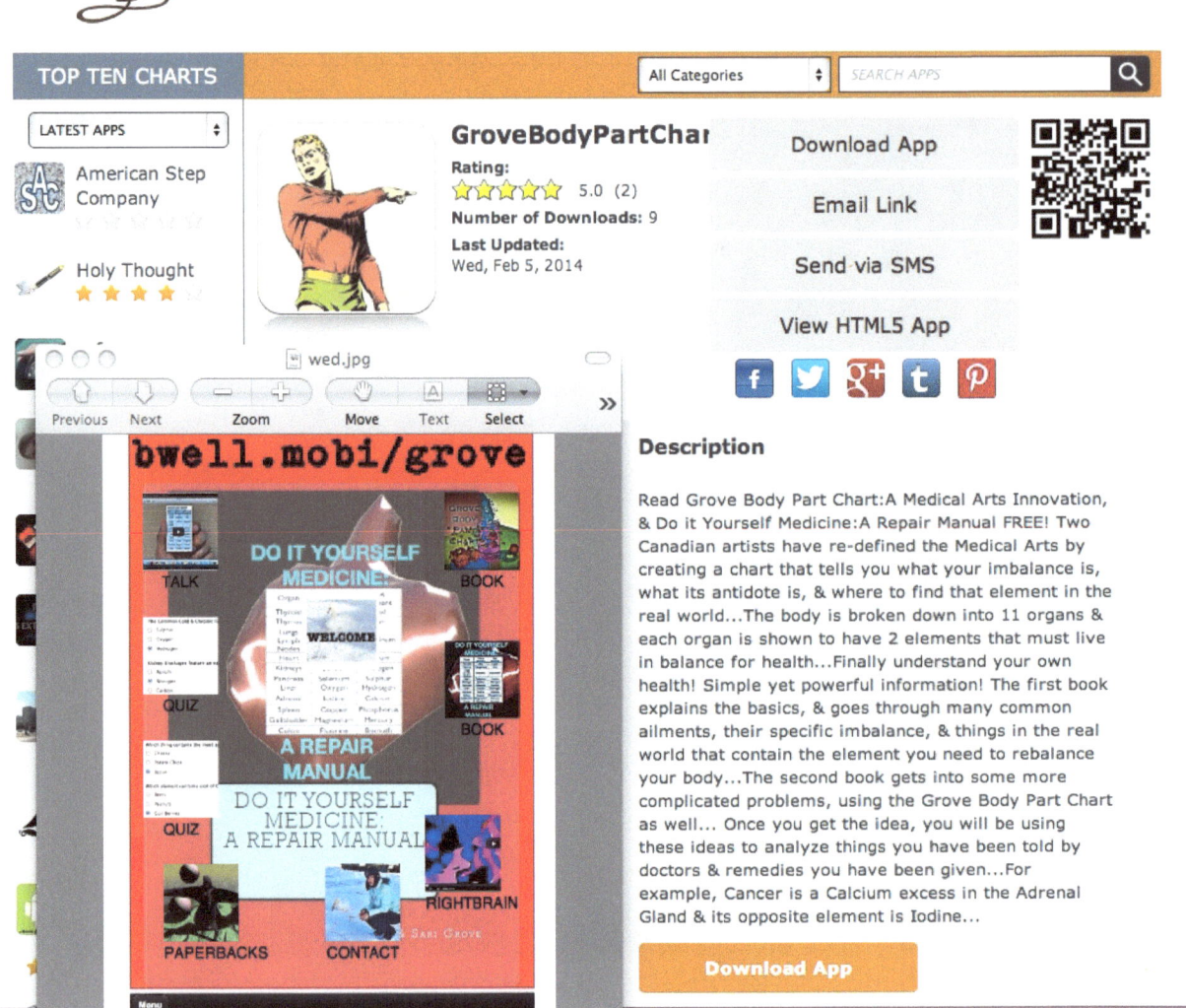

Joint pain might be bone pain...If Cortisone(Lead) shots, & laser therapy(Zinc), & Turmeric powder(Zinc from the Ginger family), are making your joint pain feel better, You might not have JOINT pain, you might have BONE pain...Because BONE involves Zinc & lead in the Thyroid Gland...So if Zinc & Lead treatments are helping to rebuild your bone & are making you feel better, you should know that your pain is deeper than JOINT pain or CARTILAGE pain, which lives in the Gallbladder & is ruled by Mercury & Magnesium...

I say this because a MISDIAGNOSIS can cause MISTREATMENT...Using the WRONG word to describe your pain might result in a protocol for that wrong word...Be very very careful what you say to people who use words like PROTOCOL...If you say Heart Attack, you may get Beta Blockers...But you might want to say really really bad constipation causing my heart to feel blocky instead...Then you get a bottle of Olive oil & instructions to add that to your daily diet...Instead of heavy duty heart meds(Potassium based) that will make you feel both puffy with fluids(anti-diuretic effect) & tired (Potassium lowers blood pressure, but so do Potassium based sweeteners like Stevia & Sugar twin & Sweet N Low & Splenda)...

What I am trying to say is...

(quote from the book Through the Looking Glass)

"When I use a word,' Humpty Dumpty said, in a rather scornful tone, 'it means just what I choose it to mean, neither more nor less.'

'The question is,' said Alice, 'whether you can make words mean so many different things.'

'The question is,' said Humpty Dumpty, 'which is to be master – that's all."

(quote from the book Through the Looking Glass)

What I am saying is that people make mistakes...Sometimes by accident...Sometimes on purpose...If there is a mistake in this book or any other of my books, please write to me ASAP & tell me what it is...or tell me in person so I can edit it out or correct it or do something...COMMUNICATE...Talk...

Communication is a very great way of solving things...When in doubt, TALK...if you have a problem, TELL...

I saw a man in a church, an empty church, in a pew, having a whole entire out loud conversation...He was talking to God...

Some people talk to walls...Walls are good listeners...

Talk...

Talk

Talk

When you are done, talk some more...

I discovered by talking on Facebook, that parenting & cleaning are linked...That having children comes with alot of cleaning...Once I knew that I felt better...I am TERRIBLE at cleaning...I would have been a terrible parent, based on the fact that cleaning & parenting are linked...This was a breakthrough for me...If you cannot even clean your own living space, the you might not be qualified to have children...No guilt...People should know that factoid..."Sorry, I cannot have children, I never learned how to clean my room"..."Oh, Ok, 'nuff said"...& they lived happily ever after...

I also found out from a site called Happify.com at http://www.happify.com that I was linking a sad event with a happy place...The Zoo...

  When Mathew Hardisty moved to California in after Grade one, it was just after we all went as a class to the Metro Toronto Zoo...For my whole life, going to the Zoo made me sad...

I am a Pioneer Beta tester(I was) for Happify...In doing the Happifying tasks, I discovered I needed to UNLINK the Zoo from the sadness of losing my grade one friend who sat in front of me & had all blonde hair...

Once I unlinked the Zoo from his leaving, I was better...Soon after, Joseph & I went to the Zoo & had the BEST time...

You have to work at being happy...Happiness is not something that just arrives like snow...Work through your sadness, UNLINK sad thoughts from happy places...

Go to the Zoo...(The High Park Zoo is mostly free)...

http://amazon.com/author/sarigrove

p.s. Arthritis can make people really mean...Fix that...Before you hurt people around you...(don't fix it with painkillers, I mean FIX it by resting & not working so hard & getting sunshine & eating shrimp & shrimp shells & eating fatty skin of chicken & bonemeal & taking glucosamine & chondroitin supplements...Fix it...Being mean is very bad for the rest of the world...Injured people tend to be mean...That is very hurtful...Be aware that if you are injured that you might be mean...So try every day to be nice on purpose...& for God's sake, fix your injury...Being sick is not attractive...It is not sexy...PLEASE please please GET WELL SOON...please...(& try to give doctors & nurses & health care practitioners a vacation by taking better care of yourself...PREVENT instead of curing...)

Skinny people need fat friends...Tendencies rub off on each other, so opposite humans need to band up too...

Banning over the counter medications like herbals means that patent holders can charge way more for new drugs based on those herbals...This is why your doctor who may be getting fed under the table by big Pharma(just a term not necessarily a bad term by the way-some big Pharma is great Pharma, some big Pharma is not-so-great Pharma), is telling you NOT to take herbals...Because herbals are a conflict of interest to the 300 thousand dollars a year on average a Physician gets who has joined the Damn Yankees team...(a film reference...Look it up)...

It is called STIRRING...You got to the veterinarian & he or she says later that a particular dog food is good for your dog & maybe sells some too you...10 years later, that veterinarian may have lost his or her inner compass & just starts telling patients that that dog food is the ONLY good one & that all the other dog foods are no good & don't buy them...STIRRING is a dangerous path for a Physician...For a politician...For anybody actually...Conflict of Interest can occur, but you shut up because you don't want the flow of money to dry up...

(Here is an example of stirring-I like the Holistic Pet Vet's book called The Stress Health Connection(it's a longer title actually)...It talks about how certain health protocols cause so much stress in & of themselves, that in the long look, not doing the health protocol is less stressful, & the dog will have a better life, untreated...This is why today, newer philosophies in medicine are to leave people alone if a treatment is mean or cruel or embarrassing & more dignity would be had with letting them live with the problem rather than carving into them surgically, or forcing them into harsh chemo protocols that kills them faster than the supposed evil tumour might have...)

DIY medicine:A repair Manual, & my first book, grove Body Part Chart:A medical Arts Innovation, come in there...There where? In between doing nothing & getting invaded by aliens...In between doing nothing & going through some pretty harsh surgeries & chemicals...Somewhere in between is a field where you do a little bit, yourself...A little bit of DIY medicine...Maybe the "Catcher in the Rye" will catch you...or God...God sometimes steps in when you give Him some time...Just because you don't believe in God doesn't mean He doesn't believe in you...I think the Holy Ghost is a more female type of aspect to the Trinity...The free liberating Wind type...The let it happen type...Let it happen...let the Spirit lead you...Sorry if this is preachy to you...Tough noogies...It's my book & I can say what I want...You don't like it, go write your own book...Then send me a link to a copy...I'll read your defense & take it under consideration...Maybe I'll even edit this tome...

Salt can kill...Salt is in the Mercury category...Salt can bring life...It all happens in your Gallbladder...In the Temporal lobe...Your lips & mouth & speech & understanding...Broca's area & Wernicke's area...Salt can make your cartilage grow & you can be an Olympic figure skater...Salt can make you dyslexic...(King Lear's daughter, the third one, liked salt...)

"A little bit of exercise is good for the body..."This is a quote from the Bible...Forget where...A little bit...A little bit...A little bit...Not...Not alot...Not...Not alot...A little bit...'Nuff said...

You can die from jaywalking...

A 19 year old son was shot in the face, lost his right eye, & part of his frontal lobe & now suffers from anger outbursts & sexual behaviour...True story...Guns are weapons...Guns are weapons...Guns are weapons...Guns are weapons...People who are weapons trained hardly ever use their guns...There are police officers who have never fired their gun during duty in their whole entire career...because they have weapons training...People without weapons training often fire their guns & sometimes shoot teenagers in the right eye causing them to lose their left frontal lobe...People with just a little bit of weapons training have fewer gun related accidents, but maybe if they were forced to have full training, we could get rid of accidents altogether...Personally I prefer a bow & arrow...or a knife...But that's just me...I also enjoy hammering coffee beans with a hammer to grind them...I like the physicality...I think gun people are lazy...A Bow & Arrow is just harder to use...Classier...

If you are missing a whole entire organ or limb or something, you need BOTH elements, MInus and Plus, to rebuild the part...For bone, you need both Zinc & Lead...For blood you need both Manganese & Iron...For muscles you need both Aluminum & Titanium...For seals & valves, you need both Potassium & Aurum...For Kidneys you need both Carbon & Nitrogen...For the Pancreas you need both Sulphur & Selenium...I explain what each organ does on an earlier chart in this book...I published two copies of the exact same chart, so the point won't get lost if you lose a page...

For the Liver you need both Hydrogen & Oxygen...For the Adrenal gland, you need both Calcium & Iodine...
For the Spleen you need both Copper & Phosphorus...For the Gallbladder you need both Mercury & Magnesium...For the Colon you need both Bismuth & Fluorine...

A defense:Indium, the use of Indium, specifically for epilepsy was pioneered in Germany...

They were using it in great dilution to control seizures successfully in the 19302 & 1940s, but that was documented stuff, they were using it before that too...

But first of all the studies are in German...WEBMD likes English studies...So if the study was in German they will just say there are no scientific studies...

It's an American conceit...if it's not in English it doesn't exist...

Also the Germans pioneered homeopathy...Americans don't like homeopathy...They also don't like Germans much...

Everything is toxic if you take too much, even water...Even Oxygen(Cyanide is just way too much Oxygen)...

Try it one night when you cannot sleep...

Hold it in your hand, put it against your skin...

What I do is I take a bar, & a nail(a good nail), & lightly hammer through a tiny hole...Do this on a cutting board...

Then take a thin stick & smooth out the edges of the hole so they lay flat...Manicure tools work...

Get a cord...Like a long leather cord, but very thin...

Put it through the hole...

Now you have a nice pendant...

Knot the ends of your cord, just with a normal double slip knot...

When you cannot sleep, put this pendant on...Against your skin...Lie down & you will sleep well & deeply...

Take it off in the morning...

Yes, too much Indium (if taken internally, which is why I like the topical methods for this), can make you feel vomity...

Melatonin is an Indium drug...Too much makes you feel vomity...But it does make you sleep & dream well...

End of defense...
p.s. Many alternative medicines are unpatentable...(No money there)...Melatonin was sort of one of them...There are partial patents...Health Canada banned melatonin...It is an Indium drug...(counteracts fluorine illnesses like epilepsy, ALS & insomnia)...But Canadians don't care...Here a red light is just a suggestion...It's like herding cats here...So melatonin is easy to get here & that's ok...But be careful...It can be addictive & cause vomiting...Maybe Health Canada & Big Pharma are not Big Brother(the book reference) but Little Sister...(me)...Before you rail against "the system" take some time to read Michael Crichton's books...Just all of them...I did...It gave me some perspective on bad people & good people...Sometimes good people blow up power stations because they didn't need more power stations in Africa because it isn't Canada...Sometimes bad people save trees...

It's all about discernment...

Sari Grove,
Sunday February 9th, 2014

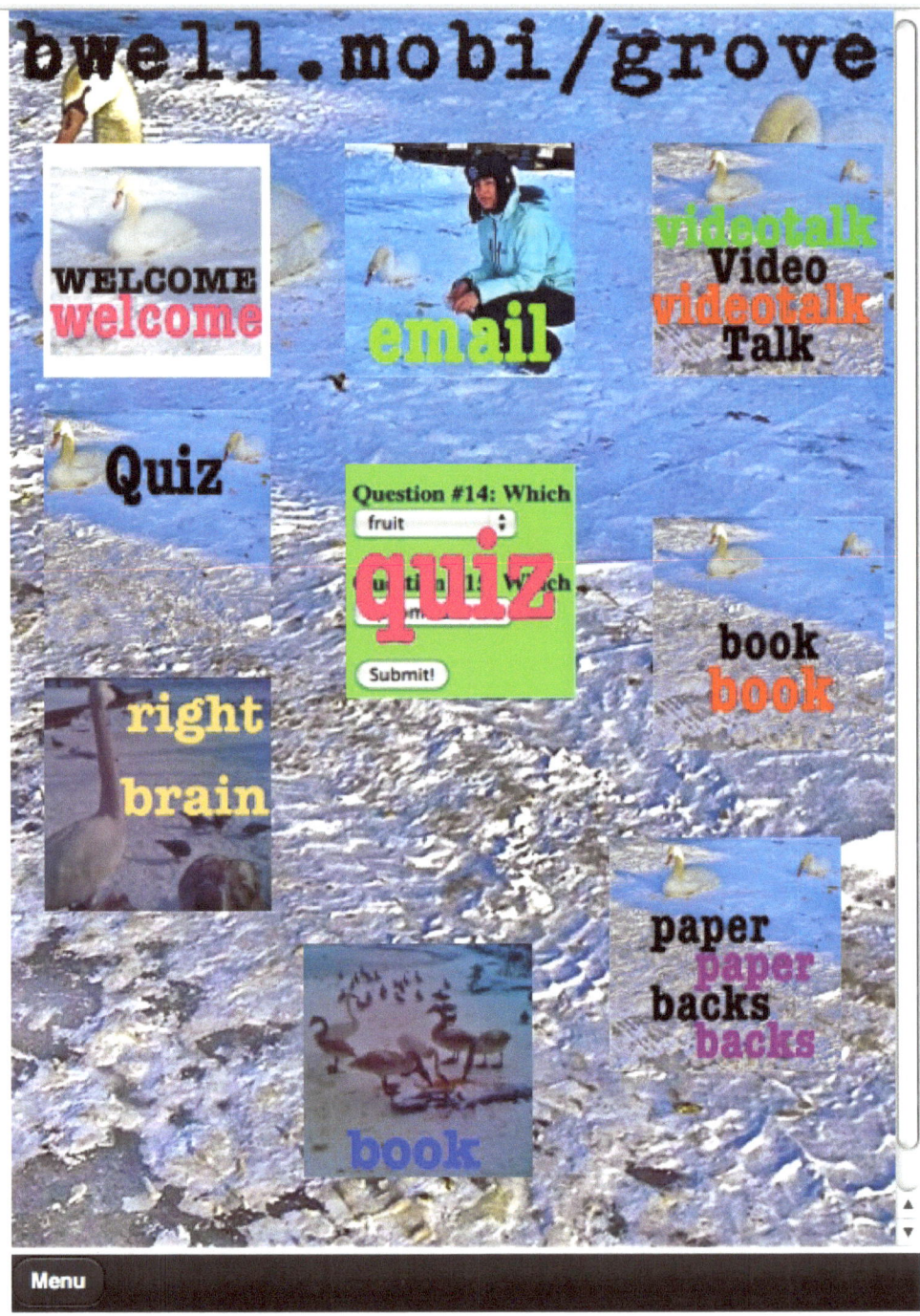

Book 3, Algae+Rhythm, Algae-Rhyme:Apt surgical rotation App, explores sidedness more thoroughly, intimating that gender is the differentiator in Brain & Body Part polarities...

www.ingramcontent.com/pod-product-compliance
Lightning Source LLC
Chambersburg PA
CBHW050848180526
45159CB00007B/2609